THE STRESS SOLUTION

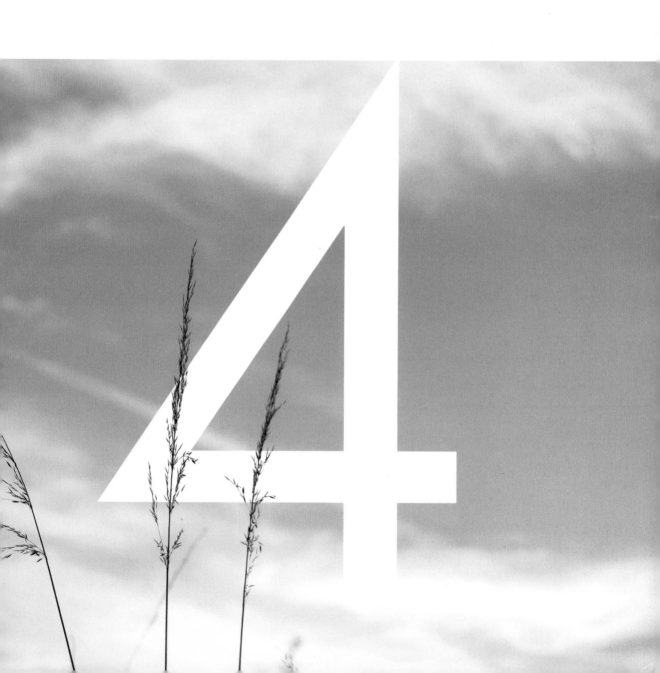

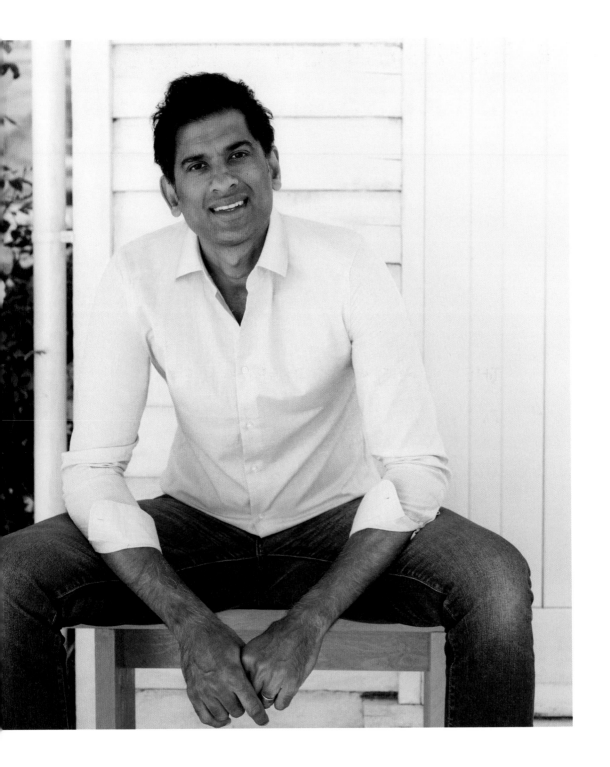

DR RANGAN CHATTERJEE

THE STRESS SOLUTION

THE 4 STEPS TO RESET YOUR

BODY, MIND, RELATIONSHIPS & PURPOSE

PHOTOGRAPHY BY SUSAN BELL

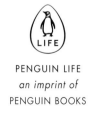

PENGUIN LIFE
an imprint of
PENGUIN BOOKS

PENGUIN LIFE

UK | USA | Canada | Ireland | Australia

India | New Zealand | South Africa

Penguin Life is part of the Penguin Random House group of companies whose addresses can be found at global.penguinrandomhouse.com.

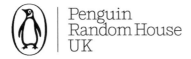
Penguin Random House UK

First published 2018
002

Set in Futura
Colour repro by ALTA Image
Printed in Europe by APPL

A CIP catalogue record for this book is available from the British Library

ISBN: 978–0–241–31794–5

www.greenpenguin.co.uk

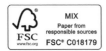
MIX
Paper from responsible sources
FSC® C018179

Penguin Random House is committed to a sustainable future for our business, our readers and our planet. This book is made from Forest Stewardship Council® certified paper.

For Vidhaata, thanks for
taking this journey with me.

CONTENTS

Introduction 8

How to Use This Book 26

1/PURPOSE 30

Chapter 1/ The 3 Habits of Calm 34

Chapter 2/ Schedule Your Time 50

Chapter 3/ How to LIVE More 68

2/RELATIONSHIPS 82

Chapter 4/ Human Touch 84

Chapter 5/ Get Intimate 98

Chapter 6/ Nurture Your Friendships 114

3/BODY 128

Chapter 7/ Eat Yourself Happy 130

Chapter 8/ Make Exercise Work For You 154

Chapter 9/ Reset Your Rhythm 176

4/MIND 200

Chapter 10/ Technology Overload 202

Chapter 11/ Bathe Yourself in Nature 216

Chapter 12/ Take Time to Breathe 230

Conclusion 254

References 256

Acknowledgements 262

Index 264

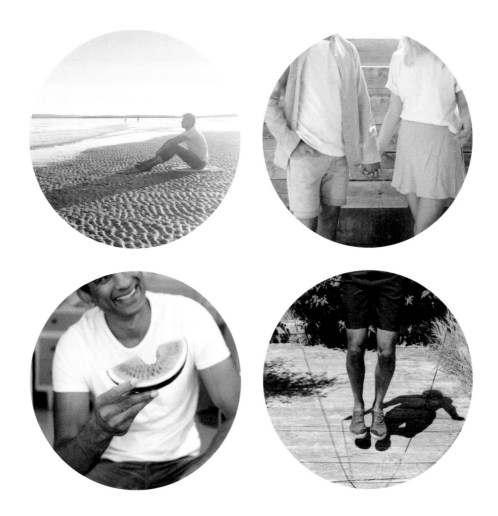

INTRODUCTION

Let me introduce you to the Cupboard of No Return. It lives on my kitchen wall. Open the door and you'll see three deep shelves, each crammed top to bottom with the shrapnel of everyday family life. Looking at it right now, I can see a golf ball, two hammers, stacks of unopened envelopes, a passport, an academic paper about mitochondria that should have gone into my previous book but didn't because it was stuffed in here, a broken screwdriver, two taxi receipts, a lightbulb that may or may not be functional, plastic pieces from a board game, a child's glove and an electric toothbrush charger. The chaos in that cupboard is the cumulative result of dozens of isolated stressful moments in the daily life of me and my young family – from when my daughter lost her glove, to when a picture fell down and I was too busy to put the hammer back in the shed, to when I was running late for work and didn't have time to put the mitochondria paper in its appropriate folder.

Here's why the Cupboard of No Return is such a problem. It isn't just the *result* of stress, it also has the power to *generate* stress. Pretty much everything in there has the potential to sprout fresh moments of anxiety and frustration – when we want to play a board game and can't find the pieces; when we're rushing to get out and my daughter has only one glove; when the electric toothbrush has run out of charge and we can't find the charger; when we're rushing for the airport and we're down one passport. Even looking at the cupboard is the cause of stress. I can feel it glowering at us as we eat at the kitchen counter, its presence a constant reminder of all the things we haven't done. Even though I may not always feel conscious of it, it's broadcasting information to my brain. It's suggesting, in a surprisingly powerful way, that my life is out of control and that there are problems in my environment that I'm just not on top of.

This is just how the stresses in our everyday lives work. The very existence of stress in our lives, minds and bodies has the power to generate more stress. The more that piles up, the less we're able to cope and the nearer we move to that threshold at which we simply stop managing our lives successfully. That's when we become overly reactive, emotional, weary and, eventually, sick. People who are stressed are more likely to fall out with others, binge on bad food and alcohol and fill up cupboards with problems that will inevitably tumble out on top of them at the worst possible moment.

THE CONSEQUENCES OF STRESS

Stress can have devastating long-term consequences for health. Too much of it contributes to the development of obesity, type 2 diabetes, high blood pressure, cardiovascular disease, strokes and Alzheimer's disease. Stress is also a key player in insomnia, burn-out and auto-immune disease, as well as many mental health disorders such as anxiety and depression.

Despite these risks, many of us are blasé about stress. We think we can get away with burning the candle at both ends for ever. The reality is very different. Every day I see patients who are literally stressing themselves to an early grave. I know a local accountant who is go-go-go the entire time. He never switches off, and his wife is worried. But because he has no serious symptoms at the moment, he won't listen to either of us. He assumes nothing's going wrong and that the stress isn't harming him. But it's probably damaging his body so much that, within a few years, I suspect he'll be hit with a serious health crisis.

Make no mistake, we are living in the middle of a stress epidemic. In fact, the World Health Organization calls stress 'the health epidemic of the twenty-first century'. Up to 80 per cent of all GP consultations are thought to be somehow related to stress. In this book I'm going to give you a series of practical solutions to help you de-stress your life. Most of them are simple and some take less than fifteen minutes a day. I've seen these tools change the lives of thousands of my patients. I know they'll do the same for you.

MICRO STRESS DOSES (MSDs)

We'll never completely rid ourselves of stress. It's unavoidable, especially in this day and age.

We're living in an era of information overload and work overload and sugar, alcohol and sitting-on-our-backsides-all-day overload. There seems to be more and more pressure on us as individuals and less and less support. Think about something as simple as booking a holiday. Twenty years ago a travel agent would have arranged it on our behalf and spared us all the hassle. Today, many of us choose to do it all ourselves, and this is the way so many things are going. We're bleeping our own shopping through at the supermarket, having to work out how to fix our own computers by digging around on baffling online forums and poring through endless FAQ lists. Particularly with the recent tech explosion, we have more jobs to do, which is creating more stress in our lives. I call such individual portions of stress Micro Stress Doses, or MSDs. Whether they come from the tech in your life or they're just the standard stresses that come with being a husband, a wife, a parent, a boss or an employee, there's not a day that goes by without you experiencing plenty of them.

Take a typical hour in the life of Alexandra, a working mum. She's had a late night and her smartphone wakes her up at 6.45 a.m. (MSD1). She flips it on and checks her Facebook feed, where she sees that a work colleague is watching the dawn on a stunning Greek island (MSD2). She flicks to a news site and sees some horrible photos taken in the wake of a mains gas explosion (MSD3) and a headline about a hate crime thousands of miles away in Canada (MSD4). She gets a text message from her phone provider telling her that her bill is ready to view (MSD5). Her husband tuts at the pinging of her phone (MSD6). She realizes she has a heavy stomach (MSD7) and a blurry head (MSD8) after last's night treat of a pizza and an extra-large glass of wine which she had allowed herself after her stress-filled day. She notices there are paw prints on the duvet as Muffles has been sleeping on the bed again (MSD9). She goes to rouse her son, who yells at her (MSD10). Feeling groggy and irritable, she yells back (MSD11). She goes to the kitchen, sees through the window that it's raining (MSD12), registers how dirty the windows are (MSD13), remembers she has to track down a plumber to check out the weird dripping noise that's coming from the hot-water tank (MSD14), has another quick look at her phone (MSD15, 16, 17, 18) as the kettle boils, sees the chocolate biscuits that are left over from last night and thinks, 'Sod it, I'm eating one' (MSD19). She realizes her son has still not got out of bed (MSD20) and, now feeling really frustrated, barks up at him to get *bloody moving* (MSD21).

It seems I'm going to have to stop Alexandra's typical hour after about eleven minutes. And if I were to list every MSD she suffers over an entire day, it would probably take up more space than I have in this book. So you get my point – MSDs are constantly flying at us from all directions, even when it seems that nothing especially stressful is happening to us. While none of us can avoid MSDs completely, this book is going to show you how to deal with their effects more successfully and, ultimately, how to orientate your life in such a way that you'll experience far fewer of them.

EVERYTHING IS INFORMATION

Taking a deep dive into stress is going to mean introducing you to a new way of thinking about life and health. During every moment of your life there's a constant interplay of information between body, brain and environment. Your brain is always monitoring what's going on with you, checking everything from your breath, to your hormone levels, to what's happening in your gut, to the things that are happening to you in the outside world. It's treating all this activity as information that's telling it what kind of state you're in. In a similar way, your gut is taking information from the food you eat, seeing if you're in a place of feast or a place of famine. Your immune system is taking information from what's happening to you physically and emotionally.

Humans exist within an *ecosystem of information*. All those sources of information talk to each other and ultimately produce just one simple question: am I safe or am I under threat? One of the big problems with the way we treat stress right now is that we often try to tackle it from a single direction. Attacking psychological stress from overwork by practising meditation or by booking and going on a break, for example, might have only a limited effect if the lifestyle choices we're making in the kitchen, or the fried-chicken shop, are generating constant stress signals in our body through our gut. In this book, I am going to tackle psychological stress, emotional stress, dietary stress, physical stress, technological stress, life stress and much, much more. My goal in *The Stress Solution* is to impact the entire ecosystem, from every direction, so that the information you are receiving is that you are safe, and not under threat.

STRESS STATE VERSUS THRIVE STATE

When your *ecosystem of information* decides that you're in danger, it switches you out of your thrive state and puts you into a stress state. When you go into a stress state, two separate biological systems are activated. The first one is called the autonomic nervous system, which controls all the automatic processes in the body, the ones we don't have to think about, like breathing and digestion. This system has two branches, the sympathetic and the parasympathetic. When the body receives information that we're in danger, the sympathetic branch releases the hormones adrenaline and noradrenaline. This sends signals to the rest of the body to actively change its functioning, for example to increase the heart rate so that more blood and oxygen are pushed out into our muscles. This is a stress state. Only when these processes go into retreat does our default parasympathetic branch – or thrive state – come back in control.

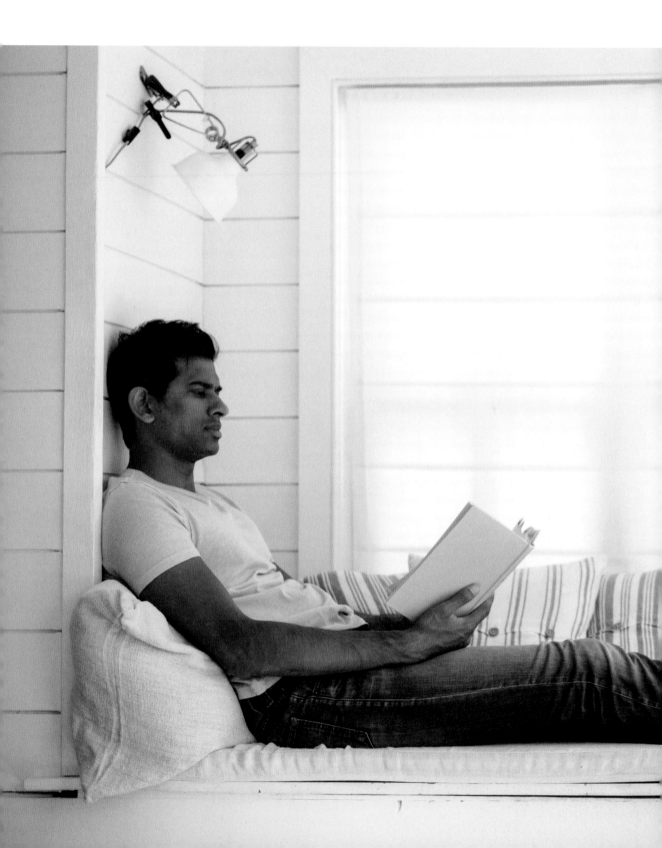

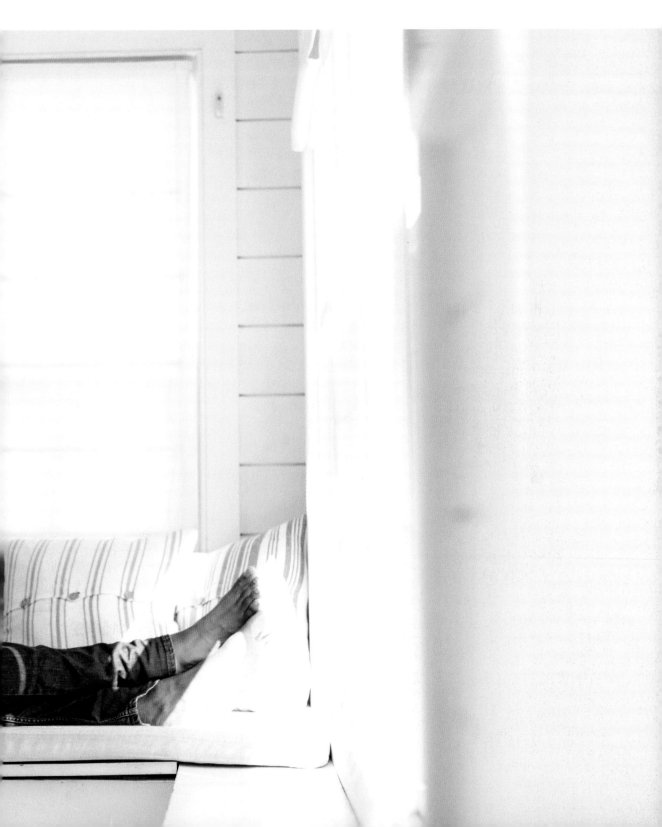

The second biological system that is activated when you are in a stress state is what we call the HPA (hypothalamic–pituitary–adrenal) axis. We can think of the HPA axis as our stress broadcast service. Stress, whether it's physical or emotional, is detected by a part of the brain called the hypothalamus. When it detects stress the hypothalamus releases a hormone that sends a stress signal to another part of the brain – the pituitary gland – which in turn releases a hormone to send the signal all the way down to your adrenal glands, which sit on top of your kidneys. Your adrenal glands then release a hormone called cortisol.

Cortisol, along with the hormones adrenaline and noradrenaline, are your body's primary stress response hormones. They put you into a 'fight or flight' state so that you're primed to deal with danger.

THE UPSIDES OF STRESS

But the stress state isn't all bad. Far from it. Your fight-or-flight response has been developed over something like 3 million years in order to protect you. Back in our evolutionary pasts we had all sorts of threats to deal with, not least the fearsome big cat, the dinofelis, which evolved to feed primarily on humans, its jaw and teeth perfectly designed for cracking adult skulls. When we were running from a dinofelis we needed to become a peak version of ourselves.

To achieve this, our stress hormones would kick into action a series of processes in the body designed to give us our best chance of survival. Our pupils would become dilated and sugars would be released into our blood so that we could run faster. At the same time, muscle and liver cells within our body would become resistant to the hormone insulin, so that more sugar would remain in our bloodstream, rather than being diverted to our muscles for storage, and thus be available for the most important organ of all, our brain. Our heart would start to beat faster and our blood pressure would rise to ensure that we could move blood quickly and efficiently around the body. Additionally, our concentration would become heightened and our brains hyper-vigilant to any possible threat. Our immune system messengers, or cytokines, would become ramped up and start sending stress signals all over our body, and our blood platelets would become activated, to prevent clotting from any injuries that might be coming our way. At the same time, our libido would plummet and our digestion would be switched off. In that moment, we didn't need to be working on digesting breakfast or, for that matter, procreating – the priority was survival. Anything deemed non-essential would be turned down or off.

And these changes would not just help us escape; if we were to get injured by the dinofelis, or had tripped and fallen during the chase, they would have been life-saving. Let's say we sustained a cut: the immune system, whose activity would have already been ramped up, would be primed and ready to help us fight infection. If we had a bleeding wound, the increased blood pressure would ensure that our brain's blood supply was prioritized over the rest of the body's and we'd be less likely to die from a haemorrhage, as our blood was more prone to clotting.

These effects are the phenomenal creations of evolution. But they've been designed to work for us only over short periods of time, as we were dealing with an immediate threat, whether it was from a dinofelis or an aggressive human being. We've evolved to live most of the time in the thrive state, punctuated by brief moments of stress. The big problem in modern society is that we're surrounded by stress triggers we haven't evolved to cope with. These continually activate the stress state, meaning we spend more time in a stress state than in a thrive state. This can have serious consequences for our health.

HEALTHY STRESS RESPONSES AND THEIR DANGEROUS LONG-TERM EFFECTS

Healthy short-term stress response

Raised blood pressure in the short term helps transport more blood to the brain

Increased blood clotting will help save your life if you have a bleeding wound, as the bleeding will stop more quickly

Increased insulin resistance in the short term means that your body won't store any sugar in your liver and muscle cells. It will result in more sugar staying in your bloodstream, which means that more will be available for the brain

The body's resources are directed at making the stress hormone cortisol to help deal with the immediate threat, at the expense of the production of sex steroid hormones, such as oestrogen and testosterone

The body's resources are directed away from digestion, as this is a non-essential function for survival at that moment

Small amounts of cortisol improve our brain function, which allows it to function better in a short, stressful situation, e.g. being attacked by an animal, or even to perform well in an exam

The emotional brain being on high alert to look out for threats is a very good thing if you are in danger

Short-term inflammation is the result of your immune system firing up to help you deal with the threat and prepares you to recover quickly in case you have a wound that becomes infected

Long-term harmful effect

Chronic high blood pressure increases the risk of many diseases, such as heart disease and stroke

Long-term tendency for the blood to clot will increase the risk of having a stroke, heart attack or DVT (deep vein thrombosis)

Long-term insulin resistance contributes to the development of type 2 diabetes, obesity, high blood pressure and the production of harmful types of cholesterol, like VLDL

Long-term diversion of resources to make cortisol will lead to hormonal imbalances and contribute to a wide variety of hormonal issues such as lack of libido and menopausal symptoms

If attention is diverted away from digestion for too long, digestive complaints will result, such as constipation, bloating, indigestion and IBS

Prolonged release of cortisol starts to kill nerve cells in the hippocampus (the brain's memory centre) and may increase the likelihood of developing Alzheimer's

If this becomes long term, it will make you more prone to anxiety, as you start to worry about everything and see danger when no danger is present

Inflammation that becomes chronic and unresolved increases your risk of most modern chronic diseases, including type 2 diabetes, heart disease, obesity and many cases of depression

SICKNESS BEHAVIOUR

Over the past few years it has become clear that chronic inflammation can be the underlying cause behind many cases of depression. Much like other stress responses, inflammation can be life-saving in the short term – for example, to help an infected wound heal – but it can start to become toxic when it is not switched off. If the body is receiving regular information that it perceives as stressful and dangerous, the inflammation becomes chronic, ongoing and unresolved, and the body starts to think it is under attack. It's long been known that one of the clever ways that inflammation fights off bugs is by making us feel tired and reducing our appetite. Back when we were evolving, weariness and nausea would have made us retreat to the back of the cave, in the dark, away from danger, encouraging us to rest until we had recuperated.

It's now theorized that many cases of depression are in fact activations of similar protective mechanisms. Some of the hallmark symptoms of depression include low mood, indifference and anhedonia (an inability to experience pleasure). In my surgery, these are some of the most common complaints. Take forty-eight-year-old Emily, who used to love walking her dogs, was extremely vivacious and self-assured. Recently, she has been coming into my surgery complaining of feeling down on herself, of lacking self-confidence, motivation and energy, having no desire to go out with her dogs, and that she no longer enjoys seeing her friends. These are the same symptoms we might experience when we're suffering from inflammation. The body reacts as if it is being attacked by a virus or chased by a dinofelis when, in fact, it is under attack from the modern world. The inflammation seems to be having a psychological effect, pushing us to the back of the cave – or under the duvet with the curtains drawn.

YOUR EMOTIONAL BRAIN

Such cases of depression will likely be exacerbated by specific changes in the brain. We have two large neurological systems which, very loosely, we can talk about as the rational brain (which makes logical decisions) and the emotional brain (which processes our feelings and fears). You can think of these systems as being in competition with each other, each one constantly vying for the top spot. Normally, when we're in a thrive state, our logical brain is in control and we can make sensible decisions. But when we're stressed our logical brain steps aside and the emotional brain takes centre stage.

This is entirely the correct response when we're in dangerous territory. It means that the brain is now hyper-vigilant for threats, which complements the physical fight-or-flight response that primes the body to react. But once the stressor has gone, the logical brain should take back control. The problem is that the brain is 'plastic' (that is, it changes its form over time), so the more frequently you feel stressed, the more powerful your emotional brain will become. The more Micro Stress Doses (MSDs) you take on, the more your rational brain will be deskilled, while your emotional brain will grow ever stronger.

The amygdala is a key component of that emotional brain and consists of two small, almond-shaped areas. They grow when we experience repeated MSDs over an extended period of time. The amygdala is an alarm system for trouble. The more it swells, the more powerful it becomes and the more sensitive it is to detecting warning signs in its environment. If your emotional brain has grown too powerful, you'll start to sense danger even when there's no danger present. The smell of a summer barbecue is misinterpreted as a house fire. A rushed email from your boss is interpreted as a prelude to sacking. An innocent glance from a friend seems sarcastic and hostile, full of hidden meaning. Your emotional brain is reigning supreme.

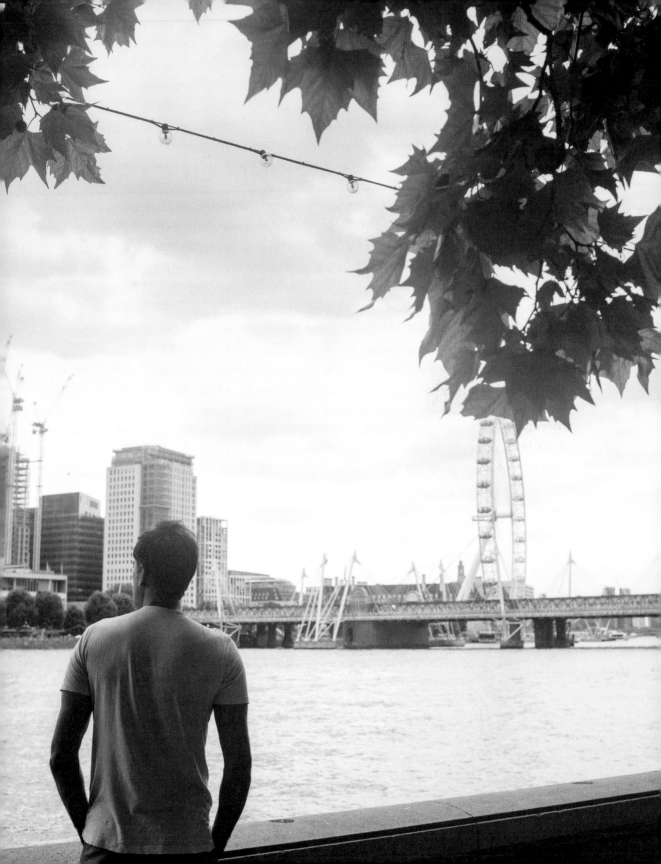

THE FEED-FORWARD CYCLE

The barrage of MSDs that modern life throws at us means that all these exquisitely balanced biological and neurological systems become disrupted. Your brain changes itself and becomes more aware of threats generally, increasing your susceptibility to them. As well as this, your stress broadcast service starts to misfire, sending alarm signals when it should be sending happy signals. Like my Cupboard of No Return, this is a feed-forward cycle. The stress you're experiencing makes you more sensitive to threat as your body and brain prime themselves against what they've decided is a dangerous environment. The more stress you experience, the more sensitive to new stresses you become. Your dominant emotional brain may make you come across as paranoid and defensive. You're also likely to make bad food choices, have less sleep and drink more alcohol. The physical stress state will begin to damage your body, as it tires of always running in fifth gear, and you may become unwell.

MACRO STRESS DOSES

While this book is primarily about dealing with Micro Stress Doses, I absolutely recognize that some people come into my surgery who've had significant Macro Stress Doses in their life – and experiences they've had in the past are impacting their behaviour, their psyche, their personality and their health. Over the last few years there's been some fascinating research carried out on what scientists call Adverse Childhood Experiences (ACEs). It's been found that people who have had these ACEs are much more likely to have various unwelcome conditions, including auto-immune disease and heart trouble. But people also suffer from Macro Stress Doses in adulthood. Some lose children, or are the victims of violent crime, or have had bad experiences while on active service in the armed forces, or some other form of adverse experience that has left a permanent mark on their wellbeing. If you're one of these men or women, I believe this book can be even more helpful to you. There's a strong likelihood that you're living your life much closer to your stress threshold than most, which means it takes fewer daily MSDs to cause you problems.

My wife, Vidh, has experienced the lasting effects of a Macro Stress Dose. When I was away for work, she used to struggle to sleep. Even though we live on a very busy street, with lots of people around, for some reason she'd become extremely scared and anxious. She'd take the kids into her room, repeatedly make sure all the doors and windows were locked and jam a chair against the bedroom door. Then she'd be up for much of the night, hyper-alert for any unusual noises. Vidh was raised in Kenya. During the coup in the early 1980s, when she was a young child, people were marauding the villages, attacking and killing people and ransacking houses. On one occasion, when intruders came to her family's door Vidh's mum put her and her brother in a kitchen cupboard and told them to be silent. Her father used to barricade the doors every evening with large sofas and heavy furniture. She doesn't consciously remember this happening, but when the story was told at a family dinner one night everyone became extremely emotional. Vidh was in tears. Once she recognized that her behaviour now was rooted in an experience that had been stamped into her subconscious, she spent time talking to a post-traumatic stress disorder (PTSD) specialist and is no longer so anxious when I am away from home. In addition, since her Macro Stress Dose is now being addressed, she is much less susceptible to all the MSDs that used to 'stress her out' because she is now living life much further away from her own, personal stress threshold.

COMFORT INSTINCTS

Of course, stress, whether it comes in micro or macro form, is nothing new. And humans are a unique animal in that, as well as our evolved biological systems, we also rely on culture to help us and shape us. Humans have been coming up with cultural treatments for stress for thousands of years, and I think it's extremely useful to look at the solutions they've come up with down the centuries with an open mind. You don't have to be a religious or spiritual person to understand the comfort that, say, prayer or practising gratitude or meditation has been for people for generation after generation. Science is just catching up with some of these and is ambivalent or even openly sceptical about others. The good news is I'm not a scientist, I'm a GP, and it's my job to understand all the latest research but also to take into account what's worked for my patients over the seventeen years I've been treating them.

HOW TO USE THIS BOOK

The Stress Solution is broken up into four pillars: Purpose, Relationships, Body and Mind. Each one represents a stress superhighway that, if you've bought this book, you probably need to get under control. In the first pillar, I introduce a big idea that is often not spoken about in the context of our health – meaning and purpose. The second pillar looks at our relationships and how the modern world is affecting them and putting them under strain. The third pillar deals with stress as it manifests in the body, in poor diet, in taking the wrong kind of exercise and keeping unhelpful daily routines. And the fourth pillar looks at our minds – how twenty-first-century living is tormenting our minds and giving us no respite, with a devastating impact on our mental health.

Importantly, each stress superhighway works both ways. A lack of meaning in our lives stresses us out, but too much stress makes it harder to find meaning. A lack of nurturing relationships causes stress, but stress itself can damage relationships. Abusing our bodies with poor lifestyle choices is a significant stressor, yet stress makes it harder for us to make those beneficial lifestyle choices in the first place. And not prioritizing the health of our minds will absolutely raise our stress levels, and vice versa. Just like the Cupboard of No Return, it's not only a result of stress, it is a source of stress as well.

In *The Stress Solution* I am going to give you practical solutions that you will be able to apply in your life immediately. Each pillar contains a wide selection of solutions that will help change the information that's being delivered to your brain and body. I'd like you to start slowly, picking one or two of the easier interventions from each of the pillars, before slowly building up. It is not about perfection in one particular pillar – you are aiming for balance across all four.

You absolutely do not need to do every recommendation. You can personalize this to what you deem most relevant in your life at this particular time. However, the more you do, the easier it becomes to do the rest. It is a feed-forward cycle, just like stress. If you are not sure where to start, pick the one thing that you feel you can do immediately and try it for the next seven days. Bit by bit, little by little, you will start to take control of all the stress in your life. You will learn how to change each stress superhighway from being a Friday-evening-rush-hour commute into a relaxing Sunday-morning drive.

The first pillar, for me, is the most crucial. I believe that the major elements missing from the lives of most people are meaning and purpose. In order to tackle this, you'll need to have periods of calm space to stop and think and then pursue one or more new activities that you are passionate about. Filling your life with meaning and purpose is the single most important thing you can do to live the life you've always dreamed of.

PURPOSE

Make Daily Affirmations
(see p. 37) ✓

Reframe Your Day
(see pp. 38–44) ✓

Practise the Three P's
of Gratitude (see p. 47) ✓

Make a Schedule
(see pp. 55, 59, 63) ✓

Zone In Each Morning: With
the Three M's (see p. 67) ✓

Apply the L.I.V.E.
Framework (see pp. 71–81) ✓

RELATIONSHIPS

Keep a Touch Diary
(see p. 95) ✓

Do the Seeing Eye to Eye
Exercise (see p. 106) ✓

Implement the 3D Greeting
(see p. 109) ✓

Make a Plan for Intimacy
(see p. 112) ✓

Become a Regular
(see p. 119) ✓

Diarize Time with
Your Friends (see p. 125) ✓

BODY

Eat the Alphabet
(see p. 144) ✓

Your Daily Exercise Prescription
(see p. 163) ✓

Burn the Stress Away
(see p. 164) ✓

Eat Your Food within
Twelve Hours (see p. 187) ✓

Reduce Liquid Stress
(see p. 190) ✓

Treat Yourself to Sleep
(see p. 195) ✓

MIND

Take a Digital Holiday
(see pp. 206–7) ✓

Mute Your Digital World
(see pp. 212–15) ✓

De-clutter Your Life
(see p. 227) ✓

Enjoy a Daily Dose of Nature
(see p. 228) ✓

Meditate for at Least Five Minutes
Daily (see p. 244) ✓

Have a Regular Breathing
Practice (see p. 245) ✓

1 / PURPOSE

When we consider stress, we don't usually think of meaning and purpose. But living a life that's devoid of these qualities is inherently stressful. I'd even go as far as to say that the single best way of living a calmer, happier life is to do it with a strong sense of purpose. But what do I mean by 'purpose'? One way of thinking about it is as living your life *on* purpose.

People with a strong sense of purpose enjoy significantly better health compared to those who don't, including less likelihood of developing heart disease, strokes and depression. Research also shows that they sleep better and live longer. Perhaps more crucially though, people with a sense of purpose live happier lives.

As a GP, I'm seeing more and more patients making good progress but then hitting a plateau. Often, when I start delving into the state of their wider lives, I find that they're not their own masters. They have no control. Things are just happening to them. The roles they've taken on in life are in charge of them, rather than the other way around. They think their job or the fact they're raising children is who they are. When I ask them about their life's purpose, they tell me, 'I'm a mother'; 'I'm a father'; 'I'm an IT worker' or 'I'm a teaching assistant.' But none of that tells me who they *really* are.

This is a crucial question that every one of us needs to ask. Are we just trying to be what other people – parents, spouses, bosses – want us to be? Or are we living our lives authentically? Do we even know who we are well enough to answer that question? If not, we need to ask ourselves, 'Why do I deal with stressful events the way that I do? Is it really me acting this way, or am I mirroring my father, my colleagues or maybe a friend I look up to? Which of these behaviours do I want to change?' These are not easy issues to tackle and you can spend your whole life trying to get to the bottom of them. But that's OK because, cliché as it is, it also happens to be true that life is a journey. Discovering ourselves is a huge part of that journey.

YOUR *RAISON D'ÊTRE*

A good place to begin is to ask what we want for ourselves. The French call this your *raison d'être*, or 'reason for being'. Ask yourself, why do you bother to get up in the mornings? Is it because you've got a list of things to do, or do you purposefully want to get up because you're keen to achieve certain things? So often, the poor lifestyle choices people make, such as bad dietary choices or drinking too much alcohol, have their deepest origins in them not being in touch with their true purpose. If you work in a job you hate with colleagues you don't like and a commute that drains and enrages you, is it any wonder that, as soon as you're back home on Friday, you open that bottle of red or peel the wrapper of that deliciously tempting chocolate bar?

I could talk to you about alcohol and sugar being bad for you, and it might make a difference for a week or even a month or two. But if drinking too much alcohol or eating unhealthily are compensation for the lack of meaning and purpose in your life, you're always going to struggle. When I hit a roadblock with my patients, this is often the underlying issue. They don't have a reason to get out of bed in the morning.

But here's the problem. In order to find out who we are and what our purpose is, and then begin to change our lives, we need time. And time is precisely the thing that the modern world is stealing from us. This was really brought home to me about five years ago as I was driving through the Dordogne region of France one Sunday on the way back from a friend's wedding. I noticed that all the little villages I was going through were like ghost towns. The shops were locked, the shutters closed; there was hardly anybody on the streets. French people, I was thrilled to discover, still protect their Sundays. They're *meaning* days, days reserved for them to interact with others, eat long meals, play in the garden and pursue pastimes and hobbies that bring them joy. Sadly, this long tradition is now beginning to erode, not least in the more urban parts of the country. If you ask me, this is a tragedy.

Thirty years ago, we had proper Sundays. We couldn't check our work emails on a Sunday. We couldn't pop to the supermarket. We couldn't jump on to some online retail site and buy things. The only programmes we could watch on TV were snooker games, Formula One rallies or black-and-white films, or so I remember. If we hadn't bought bread on Saturday, we weren't getting any until Monday. And do you know what? We coped. We managed. Now, whether it's Sundays or the continual erosion of our evenings, we're all having an essential resource stolen from us: time. There are many invisible costs to this, and one of the least understood is the fact that it robs us of the chance to really think about ourselves and our purpose in the world. We all need to feel there's a point to our existence beyond picking up a pay cheque. If we don't, we're automatically living our lives perilously close to our stress threshold.

In this first pillar I'm going to give you a selection of strategies that will help get you to a place, in your head and in your wider life, in which you can tackle meaning. Firstly, we're going to look at ways you can start seeing the life you have in a different, more positive way. This will help you achieve a mindset that's strong and calm enough for you to begin to make changes. Secondly, I'm going to help you eke out some more time in your busy day to really *think*. Then, I'm going to give you a brand-new framework so you can start the process of finding your reason to get up in the morning and your true purpose. Once you find true meaning, you will be well on your way to becoming the best, most authentic version of yourself.

And if you are one of the lucky ones and feel that you're already living your purpose or that you are well on your way to doing so, the principles I outline in this pillar will still be beneficial. They will help you to understand yourself better and to refine your journey.

Chapter 1
THE 3 HABITS OF CALM

This chapter is about setting up the practices and habits that will allow you to start shifting your mindset. It involves what I call the 3 Habits of Calm: *affirmations*, *reframing* and *gratitude*. These are simple interventions that I'd like you to try, each at a different time of the day. You don't need to do them all; they're simply tools to try in order to get going. You can use them as they are or tweak them to suit your own life and preferences. Some may appear a little scary and weird, but I'd strongly encourage you to give them a go. Once you get the hang of them, they can be incredibly helpful. They'll help get your thoughts in the right place so that you can start seeing the good that's already there in your everyday life and begin to shift your attention away from the negative (which humans have a natural tendency to do) and into the positive.

1. Affirmations

2. Reframing

3. Gratitude

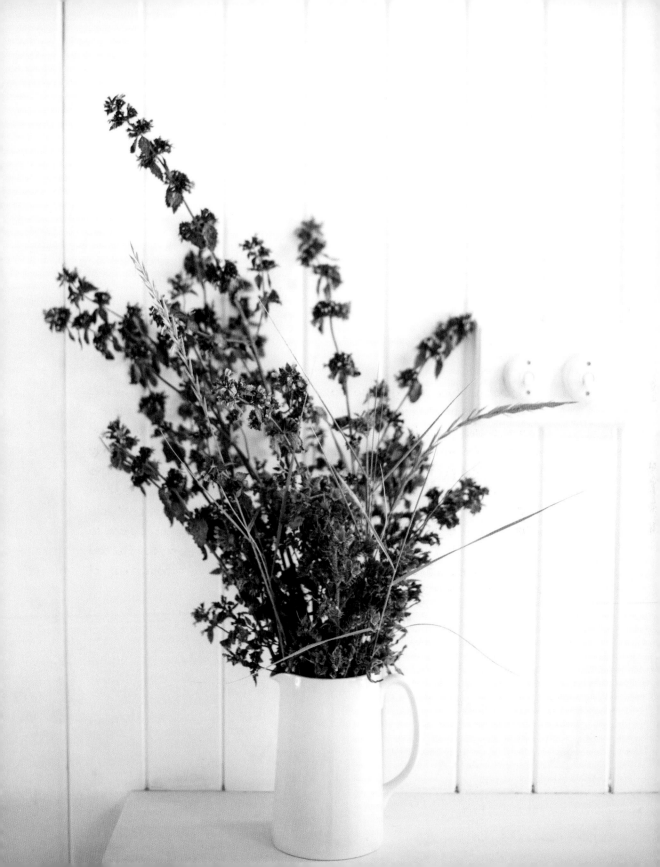

AFFIRMATIONS FOR BREAKFAST

Whether you happen to be religious or not, it seems pretty clear to me that we have a lot to learn from the gods. Every religion contains a set of guidelines that describe how to live in a way that's in harmony with those around us, good for the planet and good for us as an individual. Whether it is confession, meditation or the practice of forgiveness, many religious traditions are bristling with profound and effective *comfort instincts*. And not only religions. Many of these practices are culturally embedded all over the world.

Take my mother-in-law, who grew up in India. She's convinced that affirmations have changed her life. An affirmation is a short, powerful and positive statement of intent which you repeat regularly. 'By doing affirmations repeatedly I feel as if I'm actually changing my thoughts,' she told me. 'Because I repeat them so often, I'm laying a new blueprint in my mind.' I asked her about her rules for doing affirmations properly. 'It has to be succinct,' she said, 'because you have to repeat it as often as you can. It has to be positive. It also has to be in the right tense: it is *I am* instead of *I'm going to*.' In an affirmation, you're talking to your subconscious mind, programming in what you want out of your life. Your affirmation can be as broad as one my wife used to use – 'I am happy, calm and stress free' – or it can be more specific: 'I help my patients live happier, healthier lives.'

The brain is constantly responding to the world around us, reading it as information. The environment to which we expose our brain determines how stressed we are. Affirmations are a way of directly feeding our brain positive information, programming it for success. Regular practice will set you up for a calm, stress-free day and start changing how you see yourself and the world. If you don't believe my mother-in-law, consider this. US army soldiers who saw benefits in their deployment and agreed with statements such as 'This deployment has made me more confident in my ability' or 'This job allowed me to demonstrate my courage' were found to be less likely to suffer PTSD and depression. Affirmations have even been shown to improve problem-solving performance by undergraduate students.

SEVEN TIPS TO MAKING EFFECTIVE AFFIRMATIONS

1. **Write down your affirmation.** It should be short, as you will be repeating it over and over again, and it should also be in the present tense.

2. **Think about what you may consider to be your negative qualities,** e.g. 'I am highly strung.' An affirmation is a powerful way to flip this on its head. For example, your affirmation could be 'I am calm and stress free.' Other examples include, 'I choose to be happy' or 'I am the architect of my own health.'

3. **Experiment with different affirmations** and see how they make you feel.

4. **As you are saying the affirmation out loud, really imagine yourself as that person.** If your affirmation is 'I am full of energy' – imagine yourself as a person who is full of vitality.

5. **Say the affirmation every morning, even when you don't feel like it.** Try to do this at the same time every day to help it become a part of your daily routine. Just before breakfast or as soon as you wake up is ideal. Try to repeat the phrase continuously for about one or two minutes.

6. **Repeat the phrase as often as you can throughout the day.** This can be done silently in your head, if in company.

7. **Feel free to change your affirmations** depending on what message you are trying to imprint within your brain.

REFRAMING THE DAY

Our ability to be motivated and purposeful often depends on how we choose to interpret a stressful event. We all know that person in the office (and that person may be you) who always looks on the negative side: *Why does that always happen to me? Just my luck! Why do I never get a promotion? It's always me that's being overlooked.* The problem with this kind of victim mentality is that it tends to be self-fulfilling. By constantly thinking in this way we're training ourselves to become that negative person. We all have bad things happen to us and reasons to feel disregarded or perhaps even oppressed. But how we frame our particular situation is a choice. This framing is something we all do, all the time, whether we realize it or not. And you'll do yourself an enormous favour if you take control of how you're framing your life and make it work *for* you rather than *against* you.

There was an incredibly life-affirming example of reframing in the 2011 film *Happy*. The opening scene takes us to a slum in Kolkata, India, where we meet a rickshaw driver called Manoj Singh. He wakes at 5 a.m. and, after a small cup of tea, waves goodbye to his family. Then he slips on his flip-flops, jumps on his bicycle and pedals off to the city, where he spends a long, gruelling day on his feet, pulling clients around in his rickshaw. We learn that some customers are abusive to him, especially if they're drunk. But Manoj never complains because, if he does, they won't use his services again.

It's then that the film delivers its staggering statistic: Manoj Singh is as happy as the average American. As he pulls up at his modest home at the end of the day he has an enormous smile on his face as his young son rushes out to greet him. 'In this moment, I am full of joy,' he says. He tells us that he gets to be out in the sun each day and, if it rains, he knows it won't last long and he'll soon dry off. 'My home is good,' he adds. But his home isn't something anyone in the West would regard as good. A plastic tarp covers the roof. 'One side is open, and air flows into the room nicely,' he says. 'During the monsoon, the rain rushes in, and it does get a little uncomfortable' he admits, 'but apart from this, we live well.' Sometimes they can afford to eat meals of only rice with salt. But, he says, 'when I see my children, I don't feel as if I'm poor, I feel rich.' I found Manoj's reframing amazing. He doesn't wish he had a better job. He's thankful for having work so that he can feed his family and that he has two children to look after.

I learned about the power of reframing the hard way, when I was working at a local GP practice that had been taken over by a private company. Previously, I'd had a lot of autonomy, which is a key part of mental wellbeing. But our new owners brought in systems that took a lot of that autonomy away. They insisted on setting standard surgery opening times across all the practices they were running. But some of my patients, who I'd been seeing for years, worked night shifts and had to make appointments on the way home after work. I was very happy to arrive at work at 7.15 a.m. to see them, but my new bosses stopped me, simply because of their insistence on uniformity. Their systems began to control almost every minute of my working life. One of the managers even tried to specify exactly when we had to look through the daily blood results. Any earlier or later than the allotted one-hour window and we'd be in trouble.

This became extremely frustrating for me. I'd find myself coming home feeling wound up and stressed. The first thing I'd do after walking through the door, following a forty-five-minute commute which I'd spent in a state of toxic rumination, was mouth off to Vidh about how bad my day had been, how they wouldn't listen to me and just didn't get it … and on and on and on. I'd lie in bed all night sighing and stewing, then go back into work the next day feeling worse than ever. Vidh suggested I leave, but we had bills to pay and a mortgage to cover, so I felt I couldn't.

What else could I do? The only thing I could think of were some psychological studies I knew about that indicated people are happier when they're working in the service of others. So, I started going for a walk during my lunch break and thinking back over the morning, focusing on all the good I'd done. I reminded myself that my purpose was service. I wasn't there for myself, or my new bosses, but to relieve the pain and suffering of the people in my community. This reframing of my situation was an incredible tonic and left me feeling refreshed and energized.

There's plenty of fantastic evidence that shows we can gain huge benefits from altering the way we view our daily stresses. One 2012 study found that if we change the way we think about a stressful event we can improve our physical health and also the way our brain reacts to Micro Stress Doses (MSDs). Compared to the group who didn't, the participants in this study who reframed their MSDs had lower blood pressure, higher attention levels and even improved the efficiency of their heart muscle. When we reframe a stressful experience, not only does it feel good but we benefit from powerful physiological changes in our body. We've helped mitigate the damage that MSDs can do simply by looking at the problem in a different way.

It's important, when you're reframing, to try to focus your attention not inwardly, on yourself, but on the wider world. When you're in a stressful place, try looking at the bigger picture. Visualize yourself shooting up into the sky and seeing yourself as just another ant-like speck moving along the pavement. You're just a small part of a big world, and you're there to do some good. For example, if you're a nurse, and overworked and underpaid, try to reframe 'I'm being exploited by the system' to 'I've got the opportunity to care for all these people and help them get better.'

If you're struggling with this, ask yourself the 'three why's' of your job or primary role: Why does it matter? Why does it matter? Why does it matter? Each time you ask that question, go wider with your focus, until you reach the ultimate why. If you're a truck driver, you might answer the three why's this way: Why does it matter that I get this shipment to the supermarket on time? Because I have perishable food in the back that has to be on the shelves. Why does it matter? Because customers are relying on it being there. Why does it matter? Because they're mothers and fathers who want to feed their children, and harassed men and women who want to get home after a long day and relax over a nice meal. In just three steps, the truck driver has radically reframed his situation, transforming himself from being bored and stressed in the slow lane of the M20 into a heroic figure whose efforts will make a real difference to the lives of countless good people.

THE IMPORTANCE OF REFRAMING

When you're in the middle of an MSD swarm, your emotional brain becomes dominant and your rational brain is sidelined so you're unable to look at things logically. Without a proper, practised strategy, you're likely to spiral quickly into a whirlpool of irrational negativity. If you don't actively try to reframe the experience, you'll often find that your stress levels increase during the day as your emotional brain continues ruminating on what's happened to you and keeps finding 'evidence' that your life is a mess, that you're a victim, and that the world is unsafe and unfair. Ruminating is when you tend to dwell on situations that you find distressing or upsetting, or when you replay a problem over and over again in your mind. In the short term, it may feel as though this is helping; in the long term, it will be damaging. You will be training your emotional brain to become more powerful, which in turn makes it more likely that you will spend time ruminating in the future, and so more likely that you will become anxious.

If you're struggling to reframe your day, ask yourself the 'three why's' of your job or primary role:

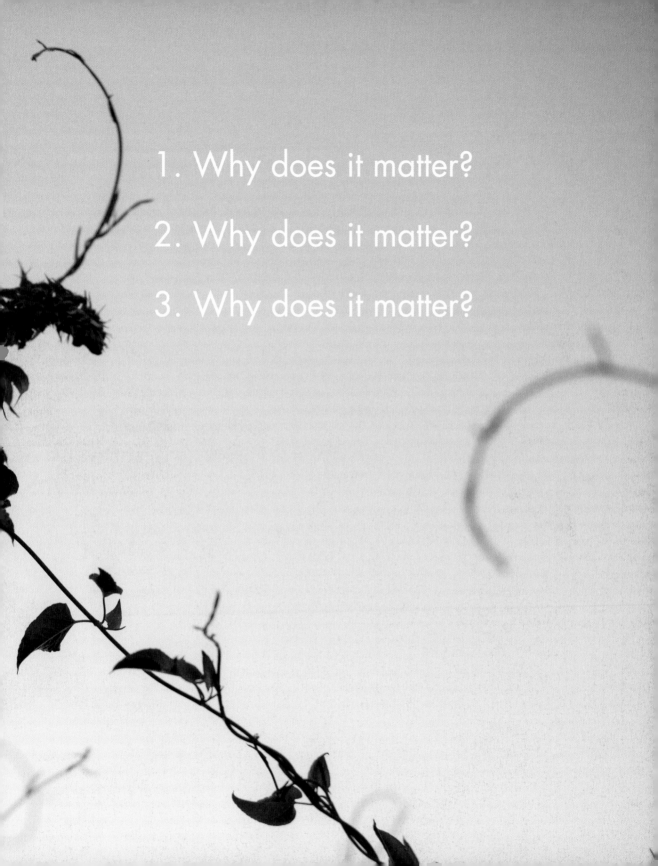

1. Why does it matter?

2. Why does it matter?

3. Why does it matter?

THREE TIPS FOR EFFECTIVE REFRAMING

1. **Write down the experience.** When we write, we tend to automatically adopt a more rational and distant viewpoint. We're able to give the situation context and clarity in a way that we can't when we replay it over and over in our head. And when we write, we tend to be kinder to ourselves.

2. **Focus on the cause.** For example, if someone cut you up while you were driving to work, instead of focusing on you and your own stress levels, try to think about the fact that the other driver may be stressed because their mother may be unwell, angry because they had a row with their partner, or has not had enough sleep because their kids were up all night. They may be on a short fuse because they left the house late and they're on a last warning at work. As soon as you focus on the other person and what might be going on in their life, you begin to put the event in context. Remember: other people's negative behaviour is evidence that they're in a bad place and that their lives are not going well.

3. **Replay the event as if you were an observer.** Reflecting on what's happened to you in the third person can often help change your perspective by putting crucial distance between yourself and what's going on. Think of yourself as a sports commentator, narrating your situation. Call yourself 'he' or 'she', or give yourself a different name. This takes you out of the heat of the moment, forces you to take a broader, less me-focused view and helps prevent you from catastrophizing.

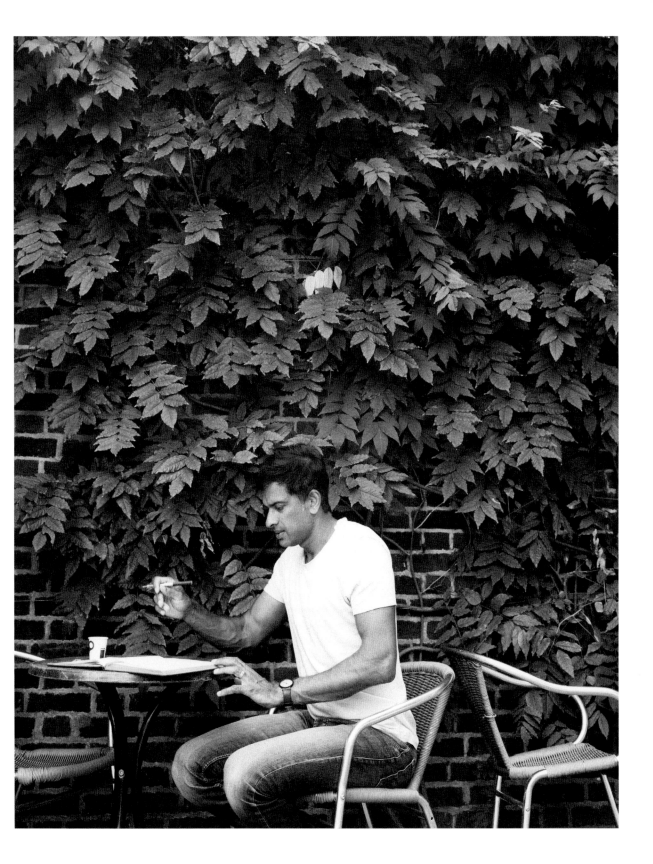

GRATITUDE IN THE EVENING

As we've learned, rumination can be incredibly damaging. Constantly stewing over stressful incidents just makes them seem worse and worse. It activates the stress state and keeps the emotional brain dominant. Gratitude is the antidote to rumination. Because we're programmed to focus on threats we miss so many of the positive things that happen to us all the time, whether it's an email we receive saying thanks for some good work or the fleeting scent of blossom as we're driving to the office.

This intervention is partly inspired by the practice of 'loving kindness' meditation. This type of meditation comes in many forms, but what they have in common is that they help develop goodwill, warmth and kindness. For instance, you might identify two people you know and purposefully wish them happiness. Or you might pick two people you don't know. Next time you're sitting in a café, identify a couple of passers-by and really try to wish for them to be happy, then observe how you feel.

A daily practice can have profound knock-on effects. Studies have found it can trigger a wide variety of positive emotions, including love, joy, gratitude, contentment and hope, as well as reducing the activity of the emotional brain. I was delighted to read a recent analysis of the published research in this area which concluded that 'loving kindness meditation can enhance positive emotions in daily life'. The scientific research backs up what I have seen in my consultation room over many years.

One of my patients, forty-two-year-old Sophie, found this kind of meditation life-changing. She had been suffering from panic attacks for a little while and was struggling to get any relief. I persuaded her to give this form of meditation a try. She decided to do it at the school playground after dropping her kids off, picking two other parents, one she liked and another she didn't. She'd use her whole mind and body to sincerely wish them happiness. A few days into the practice, her husband said, 'What is up with you? You seem to be happier these days, you've got a real spring in your step!' Over the coming weeks and months, she experienced less stress and her panic attacks became much less frequent.

If these practices don't sound like they'll have any effect on you, I challenge you to give them a go. They're really hard to do without starting to smile. You'll feel good about yourself, your focus will be pointed outwards and your stress levels will plummet.

PRACTISE THE THREE P'S

A daily practice of gratitude is a fantastic way to lower your stress levels. You can do it at any time of the day but the evening can be a particularly effective time. It can really help to lower your stress levels, helping you switch off and fall into a deep, relaxing sleep.

My own remixed version of loving kindness meditation involves spending just a few minutes at the end of each day projecting gratitude towards the three P's:

PERSON. PLEASURE. PROMISE.

Think of a person you feel grateful towards that day and, with all the power you can muster, focus on wishing them gratitude. Then do the same, but towards a pleasure you experienced during the day. Whether it was a lovely cup of coffee or a precious new memory you made, with one of your children perhaps, bring it back to life in your imagination and flood yourself with a powerful feeling of gratitude. Finally, think about something that popped up in the day that held some promise for the future. It could be setting that date to meet up with your friends, something you hope will happen at work, or even a new pair of shoes you intend to buy. Imagine that promise of the future really happening and, once more, focus powerfully on feeling gratitude for the hope that it's brought you. If you want to significantly magnify the power of this intervention, write down the things you feel gratitude towards.

ONE STEP CLOSER TO PURPOSE

This chapter is all about getting you in the right mindset to find your purpose. The 3 Habits of Calm – *affirmations*, *reframing* and *gratitude* – will help you significantly reduce your stress levels and put you in the right frame of mind for tackling the big questions of meaning and purpose. In order to do that, though, you'll also need something else: time. This is the subject of the next chapter.

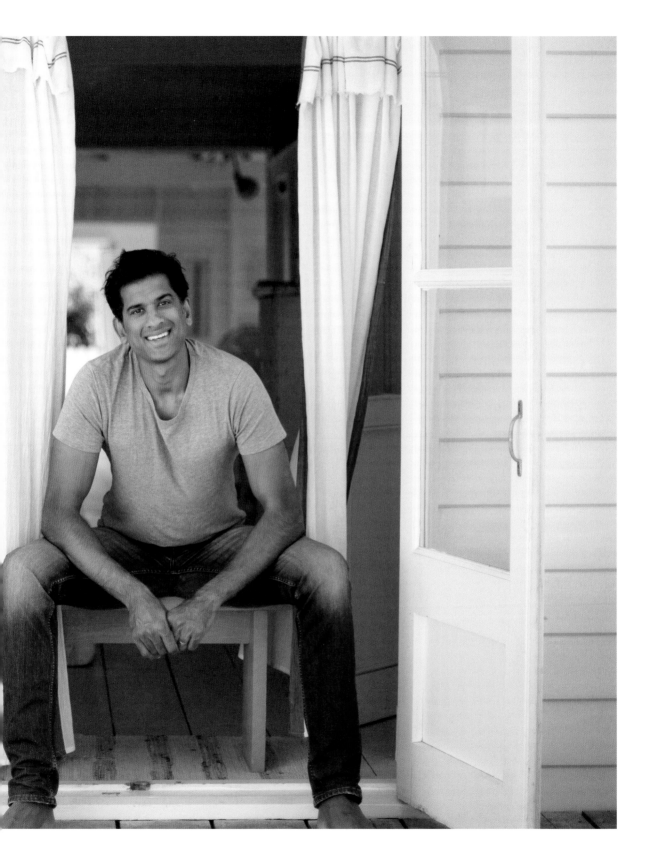

Chapter 2
SCHEDULE YOUR TIME

My wife used to be a successful criminal barrister. At the age of thirty, she decided she wanted to devote her time to being a mother so she made the decision to give up her career temporarily. We were both shocked when it became apparent that raising children left her feeling more stressed than the high-powered legal work she'd been doing for years. One thing that made her particularly anxious was the feeling that there wasn't enough time in the day. She'd take our son to nursery, and by the time she'd come back, cleaned up, done the washing and popped into town to complete all the jobs that needed doing there, it was time to pick him up again. It just went around and around like this, day after day, and the relentlessness of it all would crush her. 'I just don't get any time to myself,' she'd keep saying. 'I don't get anything done.' This, I now realize, is not an uncommon problem. I've observed it in my practice and also in my own friendship network: incredibly bright, driven and successful women and men who decide to give up their careers to raise children, only to end up suffering with anxiety.

Vidh and I began hunting around for something that would stop her feeling this way. I'd love to tell you that it was me who found the solution, but it was my brilliant wife. She started making a detailed daily schedule that accounted for every single minute of the day. She wrote down: 'Wake up: 6.30, Get ready: 6.45–7.05, Breakfast: 7.05–7.25,' and so on, like this, all the way through until bedtime. This seemed pretty intense to me. Surely this would build anxiety rather than lessening it? But Vidh found that it worked. She felt more in control

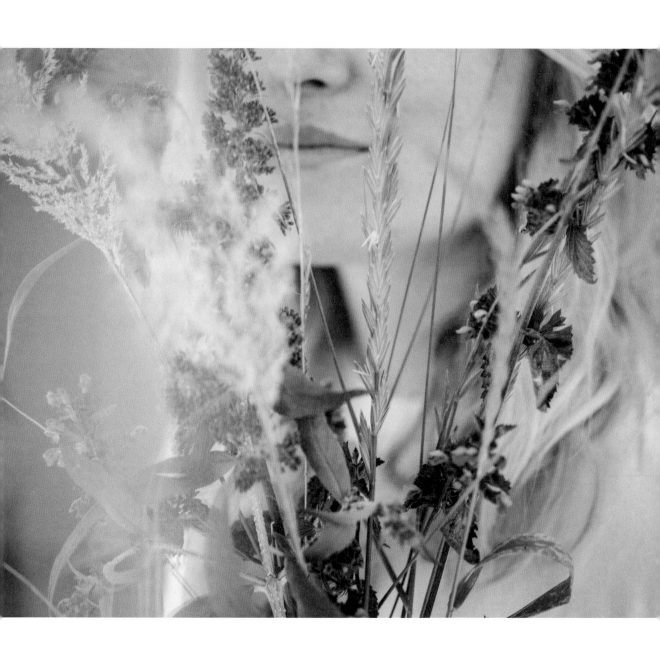

of her life. She was able to get more things done and at the same time felt fully able to enjoy the time she had scheduled for herself, to practise her yoga, and even to spend time surfing the internet, without feeling any guilt. Whereas she used to think she wasn't getting anything done, she would now see a long, satisfyingly ticked list in her A4 notepad at the end of every day.

In some ways, humans are quite simple creatures. We're wired to get a little dopamine buzz from completing tasks. We love that feeling of ticking even tiny achievements off, reminding ourselves that we've done something. Just by making that tick with the pen we make some positive information for the brain: we're in control of the day and life is good. But Vidh's practice of scheduling had an even bigger impact than that. She started to beat her own schedule. She began to enjoy doing so, almost as if it were a game she was playing against herself. She quickly found gaps opening up in her daily diary that hadn't been there before.

I've since learned that many top CEOs around the world use scheduling for this reason. It helps them be more productive, while ensuring they have ample time to pursue hobbies as well as spend time with their families. If you're one of the many people who feel there aren't enough hours in the day and that they never get enough done, take a good hard look at how you spend your day – I expect that, if you did a brutal analysis of your day, you'd probably be shocked to find how much time you've whiled away on social media, email or just prevaricating until you have no choice but to get on with things. Of course, you may also find that you really do have too many jobs to try and fit in within a short timeframe. Scheduling will also address this: it will help you prioritize the most important things that you need to do, improve your efficiency and help you find time to do more of the things you love.

If you feel you don't have sufficient meaning and purpose in your life, scheduling is critical. Let's say you want to be a writer. You're going to give it a proper crack – but only when everything's perfect: when you have a couple of hours completely free, when you're feeling inspired, when the house is quiet, when your partner's mess is off the kitchen table. This is never going to happen. That moment does not exist. It's why you need to get into the practice of writing every day, no matter if the muse isn't with you or the house is noisy – and then you'll find that inspiration will come. Instead of waiting for yourself to *feel* right, you need to purposefully schedule that action in.

Throughout this chapter, I am going to ask you a series of questions and suggest a whole array of strategies to enable you to free up more of your time. These strategies will ensure that you can do more of the things you love, feel less stressed and find precious time to be alone and think. I will also share an extremely effective technique that will enable you to start off each day a million miles away from your personal stress threshold and primed for meaning and purpose.

'DO' TIME, NOT 'ME' TIME

Within just three weeks of beginning her daily scheduling, Vidh found she had enough free time to begin a hobby that she'd always fancied trying: indoor climbing. She'd go to a local centre twice a week and come back like a different person. When she was on the wall for those two hours she was concentrating so hard she was unable to think about the hassles of her daily life. This was a form of pleasure inherently different from relaxing on the sofa or mucking about online. This was not 'me' time, it was 'do' time. When we're doing something purposeful and actively absorbing, our attention is forced away from our troubles. For Vidh, climbing had the additional benefit of being something she hadn't tried before: research shows that it is new experiences that really help the brain grow, by activating different pathways, which in turn also helps it shift out of stress state.

THREE QUESTIONS TO HELP YOU SCHEDULE

1. **Which activity would you love to spend more time doing,** something you feel you can't find time for in your daily life?

2. **What are the three most important things you want to get done** on any given day that would make you feel as if you have 'won' the day?

3. **Which person (or persons) would you like to spend more time with than you currently do?**

The best way to achieve these things is to schedule them in. You don't need to strive for perfection – just thinking about these things and starting to schedule a few of them in will make a big difference.

THE HEALING POWER OF SOLITUDE

There was also another benefit to Vidh's new pastime. When she was up there on the climbing wall, she was all alone. She was given the space to think. One of my favourite quotes is from the Pulitzer Prize-winning poet Carl Sandburg:

'*A man must find time for himself. Time is what we spend our lives with. If we are not careful we find others spending it for us . . . It is necessary now and then for a man to go away by himself and experience loneliness; to sit on a rock in the forest and to ask of himself, "Who am I, and where have I been, and where am I going?" . . . If one is not careful, one allows diversions to take up one's time.*'

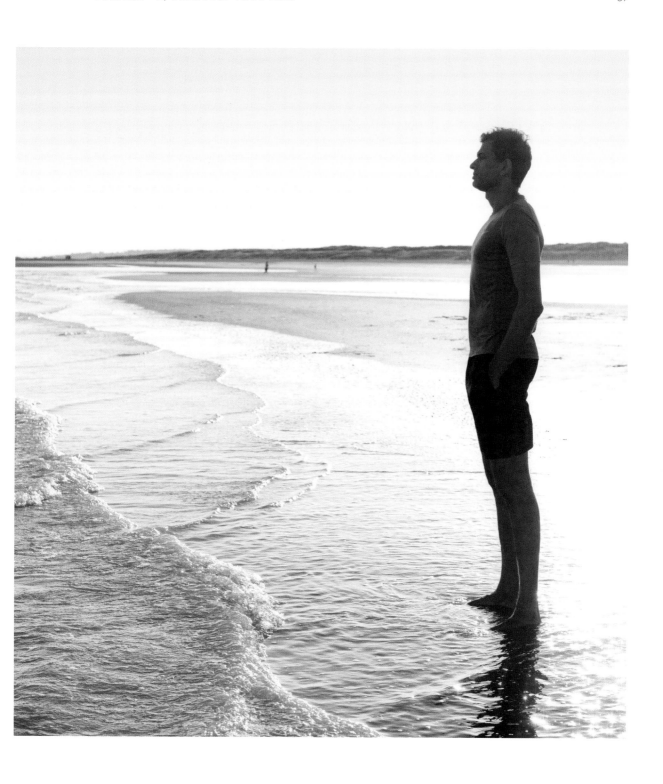

I learned this lesson for myself in the months following the death of my father. For many years beforehand, I'd been his carer. I had a young baby, a wife and a busy job as a GP, and every instant I had outside those things was spent doing things for my parents. My phone was never off; I'd sleep with it beside my pillow. I was always waiting for the call: 'Dad's fallen, can you come round and help?'; 'Dad can't get out of bed, can you come and get him out?' I was stressed out to the max. Every little thing – a difficult patient, a problem with the kids, a dish being out of place – would bother me because I was way over my stress threshold. I just had no capacity left.

After my father passed away I found I had space. For the first time in my adult life I began to sit and reflect. I realized that, for years, my life had been going at a hundred miles an hour and I hadn't had the time to work out who I really was. From the moment we're born we're placed on this very specific and narrow ladder of perceived success. We're told by our teachers and parents, 'You have to do well at school and, if you get good grades, you're going to get a good job, and then you'll live happily ever after.' We're also told that we need to marry and have the perfect nuclear family in order to be happy.

Many of us, myself included, tick these boxes which society promises us are meaningful, only to wake up one day and realize that we've been conned. This was true for me, and it may well be true for you. This is what downtime is for: to empty the mind of the noise of the outside world and fill it up with yourself so you can start working out exactly who you are. The time I spent doing nothing but thinking was the start of me living a more purposeful, authentic life.

THREE THINGS TO SCHEDULE THAT
WILL REDUCE YOUR STRESS

1. **Something that brings you joy.** It could be anything that gives you a daily dose of pleasure, such as five minutes of dancing when you get home, or listening to music. Chronic stress makes it harder for the brain to experience pleasure, so bulletproof yourself against this with a daily pleasure hit.

2. **Something that trains your ability to delay gratification** (see p. 210), such as taking up a new sport or hobby, or learning a new language or to play a musical instrument.

3. **Something that involves movement or exercise.** This can be a five-minute bodyweight workout or an hour-long class in the gym. There are no rules, but scheduling it in as an unmoveable part of your day will ensure that it happens.

STARING AT A TREE

One of the big problems with modern culture is that it associates 'busy' with 'successful'. We like to feel our schedules are full to bursting because it makes us feel that we are in demand and important. There's also a pernicious idea out there that to really excel in life we need to give all day, every day, over to our ambitions. Well, tell that to Armando Iannucci, a man who's not only had a long career as one of Britain's greatest living satirists but has broken America with his hit sitcom *Veep* and films such as *In the Loop* and *The Death of Stalin*. 'I refuse to work evenings or weekends,' he told one newspaper. 'If a script sees my character meeting for dinner, I put a line through the words and make them meet for lunch. After 6 p.m. I turn my phone off. I told the Americans I don't do calls after then.' And what does he do with that time? 'I really like to indulge in the doing-f**k-all thing. You know, just stare at a tree or something.'

He's possibly a smarter man than he realizes. Iannucci might not be aware that 'just' staring at a tree can be incredibly productive. We think the brain 'switches off' or 'disengages' when we're not focused on completing a task. This is not true. When we 'switch off', a system in the brain called the default mode network (DMN) goes into overdrive. The DMN is a powerful source of idea generation. It's why people come up with their best ideas in the shower or when walking the dog. Perhaps the secret of Iannucci's incredible creative success is his ironclad insistence on scheduling regular downtime.

I know you're busy and under pressure, as we all are. But if Armando Iannucci can do it, I humbly suggest you could too. Ultimately, 'busy' is a choice that we make. You've not *become* busy, you've *done* busy. And I totally get it – I also do busy: I struggle with this problem really badly. What I've found is that, when I protect my own time by having a strict schedule, I'm infinitely more productive for the rest of the week. I'm happier. I feel calmer. We delude ourselves that we can continue working and keep going every single day, without consequence. We can't.

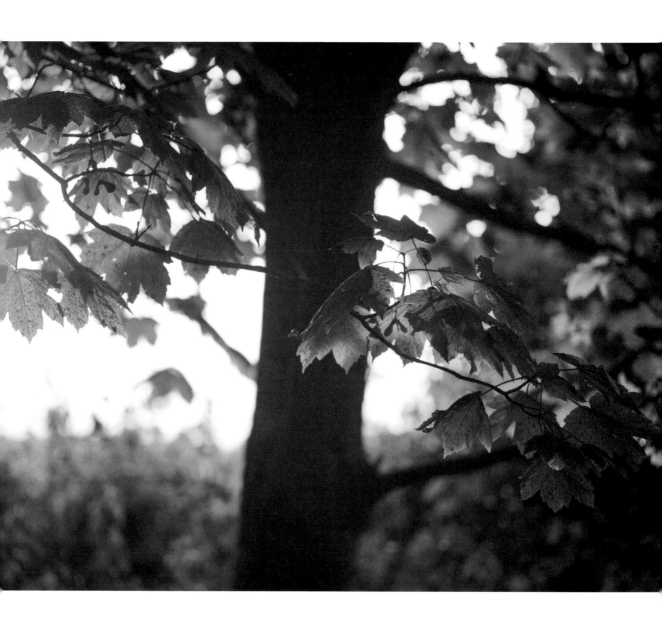

THREE TIPS TO HELP YOU FEEL LESS 'BUSY'

1. **Protect some 'me-time' every single day.** This can be as short as ten minutes but, by scheduling it in, it is much more likely to happen. It could be a quick walk in the park, a few minutes of deep breathing or simply sitting in a café watching the world go by.

2. **When you are feeling stressed on a busy commute, why not try listening to an inspiring podcast or some relaxing music, doing a bit of meditation with an app such as Calm or focusing on some deep breathing.** You will immediately take your mind away from being 'busy' and into a more relaxed and calm state.

3. **Next time you are in a queue for something, e.g. at a café or the supermarket, try to do nothing.** Don't jump on to your smartphone to check emails or social media. We are constantly filling our brains with more and more things whenever we get a moment of downtime. Try to be present with all that is going on around you and use it as a mini-moment of calm. Just be.

These practices will shift your brain from stress state to thrive state.

SCHEDULE YOUR ENTIRE DAY

I highly recommend that you try, at least once, to schedule your entire day. Put in absolutely everything you need to do. Ideally, you would continue this practice for an entire week. It is common for people to find that this practice enables them to get more things done than they thought they had time for. It is a great practice to try, even if you end up toning it down afterwards to scheduling in only the most important parts of your day.

It is critical that you schedule in your 'free time' as well as the tasks you have to complete. This may seem a little prescriptive, but I assure you that you will find this practice will unexpectedly give you much more flexibility to do the things you love!

As a bonus, at the end of each day, go through your entire schedule and see how much of your day is spent doing things you 'have to do' versus doing things that give you meaning and purpose. Try to start shifting the balance towards the latter.

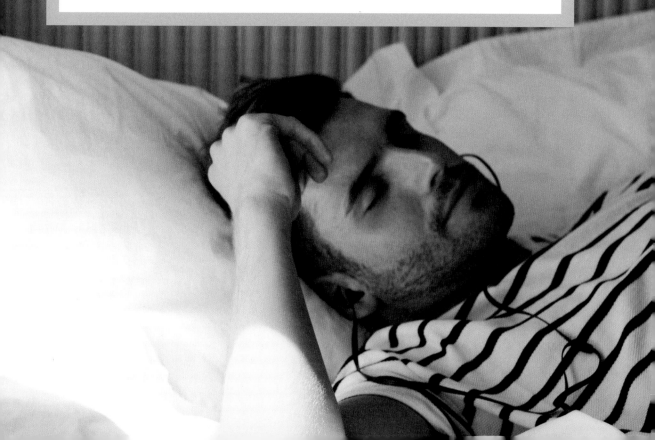

ZONING IN

If you think that diving straight into full-day scheduling might be too much, I'd encourage you to at least practise having a regular morning routine which helps you to 'zone in' for the day. This is one of the best methods I know for sending rivers of thrive information into your brain and body. It's crucial to understand that your actions create your mood. The very act of putting yourself through a series of familiar, habitual steps at the same time every day tells your system that you're in a place of safety and control and helps shift you into thrive state at just the right time. The things you choose to do as part of your own personal ritual will add layers and layers of bonus benefit on top of the routine itself.

One of my patients found an unexpected cure for her skin condition in her morning routine. As well as eczema, thirty-seven-year-old Victoria suffered from anxiety. She noticed that her eczema would flare up when she felt stressed. On one occasion, she ruefully commented that it was 'reacting to her life' – in other words, reacting to the stresses, resentments and the absence of meaning in her never-ending to-do list and the lack of control she felt over her life.

Victoria would wake up as late as she possibly could. Her alarm would be blaring, the snooze button hit four or five times. Then she would be go-go-go from the minute she woke up. She started each day in a stress state perilously close to, if not past, her personal threshold. I tried to persuade her to work to a morning routine as soon as she woke up, but she resisted the idea. She felt it wouldn't work for her. She had two children, aged seven and nine, who she needed to get ready for school. Eventually, I convinced her to wake up ten minutes earlier and put a routine in place that appealed to her. She decided to light a candle, spend three minutes doing alternate-nostril breathing (see p. 241), three minutes doing the Sun Salutation yoga sequence and two minutes saying affirmations (see p. 36).

In all, it would take just those ten minutes, and by keeping the bar low she managed to achieve it every day. Once she had finished her morning routine, she would wake up her kids and carry on as usual. She told me that her mornings immediately felt less stressful. And not only did her skin condition improve, after six months she felt centred enough to start making bigger changes in her life. Not a bad result for an investment of just ten minutes per day.

MAKING THE TIME

I appreciate that not everyone will feel that they can zone in first thing in the morning. It is important to find a time that works for you. Some of my patients with children end up doing a 'zoning-in routine' for ten minutes in the car after they have dropped their kids off at school or once they have returned home. Some patients do it outside their workplace before they go in. My own personal belief is that first thing in the morning is best, as it sets your body and mind up for the day, but start in whatever way you can.

For me, zoning in each morning makes all the difference in the world. It primes my body for the day ahead and I'm still reaping the benefits in the evening. But if I wake up a little late and I don't get time to do it, or if I feel a lack of motivation and jump on to Facebook or email instead, it's completely different. I start the day much closer to my personal stress threshold. As much as I value sleep, I'd argue that getting up ten or fifteen minutes earlier to give yourself some time and space in the morning is more important. It shifts you from being in a reactive mindset to being in a proactive one. What you do at the start of each day sets up the way you live that day, and those individual days build up into a whole life – a life lived on purpose and a life lived *with* purpose.

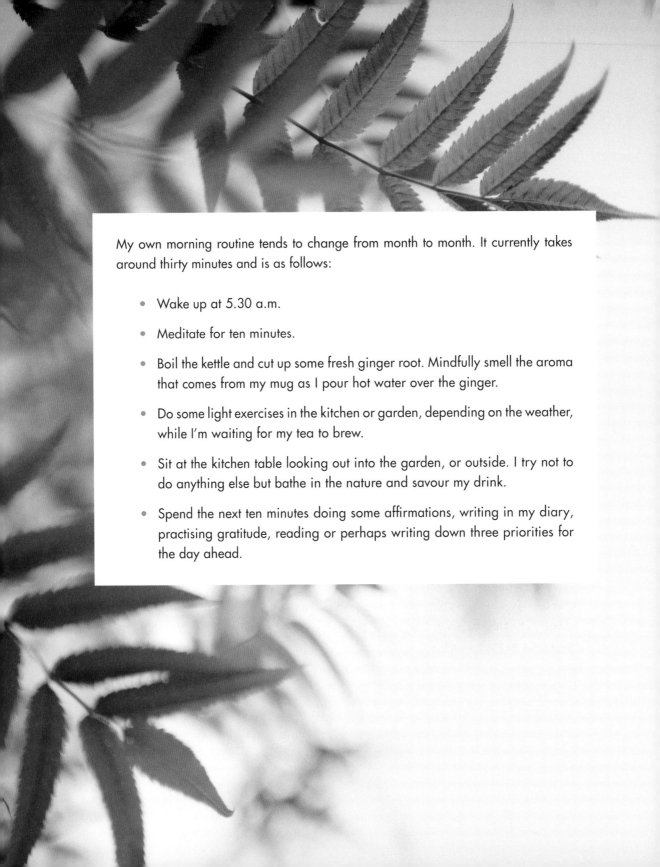

My own morning routine tends to change from month to month. It currently takes around thirty minutes and is as follows:

- Wake up at 5.30 a.m.

- Meditate for ten minutes.

- Boil the kettle and cut up some fresh ginger root. Mindfully smell the aroma that comes from my mug as I pour hot water over the ginger.

- Do some light exercises in the kitchen or garden, depending on the weather, while I'm waiting for my tea to brew.

- Sit at the kitchen table looking out into the garden, or outside. I try not to do anything else but bathe in the nature and savour my drink.

- Spend the next ten minutes doing some affirmations, writing in my diary, practising gratitude, reading or perhaps writing down three priorities for the day ahead.

ZONE IN EVERY MORNING: THE THREE M'S

When designing your routine, you can choose interventions from any section of *The Stress Solution*. It can be as short as five minutes or as long as an hour. You'll want to cover three broad bases, which I call the three M's:

MINDFULNESS: This will give you an immediate short-term shot of calm. Think breathing, being in nature or meditation.

MOVEMENT: You'll want to prime your body physically. Think skipping, t'ai chi or yoga (see p. 166 in the chapter on exercise for more details).

MINDSET: Send your thoughts in a positive direction. Think gratitude, affirmations or loving kindness meditation.

It is good practice to have a golden hour each morning without your mobile phone on. By doing this, your mind will continue to process what you dreamed about the night before, rather than being jerked into the horrible realities of news and social media. Allow it to wander and you will often come up with some super-creative ideas, whether they are for work, play or lead you towards solving nagging problems in your wider life.

Chapter 3
HOW TO LIVE MORE

Two summers ago a CFO of a local plastics company came to see me in my surgery. Simon was in his early fifties, was feeling stressed and depressed, and had been for at least eighteen months. His diet was fine, without being amazing, but his job was unrewarding and taxing. As we were talking, I asked him if there was a hobby that he had enjoyed doing when he was a boy. He looked slightly uncomfortable before eventually admitting he had enjoyed playing with an electric train set. 'Do you still have it?' I asked.

'Oh God, I don't know.' He smiled and thought for a moment. 'It's in boxes up in the attic somewhere.'

'I wonder if you could do me a favour?' I said. 'Get it out on Sunday. Set it up and see how you feel.'

He took the suggestion surprisingly well but never came back to the surgery for a follow-up. I managed to find out what had happened only by chance, a few months later when I was leaving my surgery to do a home visit and I crossed paths with his wife in the car park.

'He's getting quotes for a big shed at the bottom of our garden. I've never seen Simon so excited,' she said. 'It's for his train set. He's obsessed with it.'

'Really?' I said. 'That's amazing!'

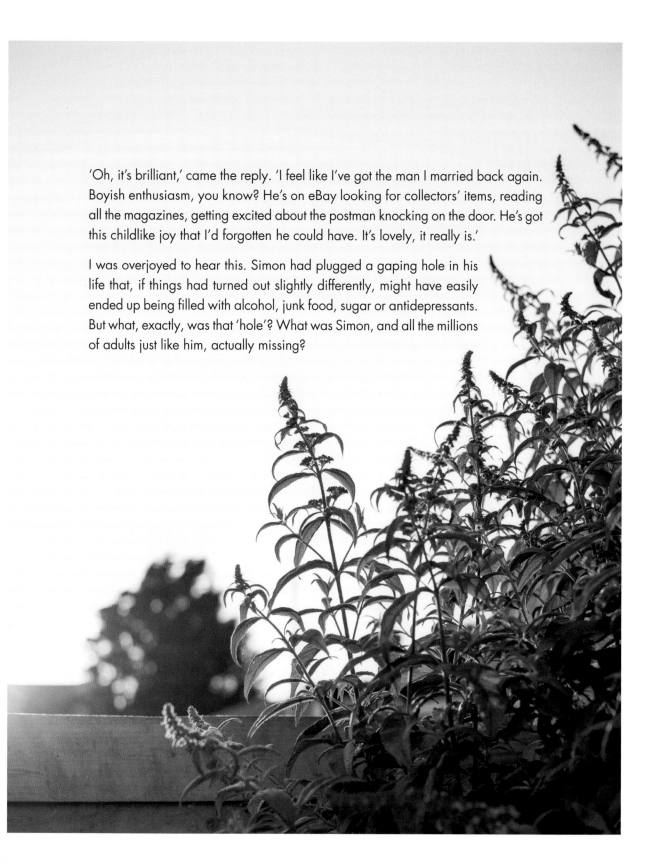

'Oh, it's brilliant,' came the reply. 'I feel like I've got the man I married back again. Boyish enthusiasm, you know? He's on eBay looking for collectors' items, reading all the magazines, getting excited about the postman knocking on the door. He's got this childlike joy that I'd forgotten he could have. It's lovely, it really is.'

I was overjoyed to hear this. Simon had plugged a gaping hole in his life that, if things had turned out slightly differently, might have easily ended up being filled with alcohol, junk food, sugar or antidepressants. But what, exactly, was that 'hole'? What was Simon, and all the millions of adults just like him, actually missing?

IKIGAI

This is a profound and complex question and goes to the very roots of the human condition. One compelling answer to it can be found in Japan. There, they'd be likely to say that Simon had been missing his *ikigai*. The word *ikigai* comes from *iku*, meaning 'to live', and *gai* which means 'reason'. While it may sound similar to the French concept of *raison d'être*, there's actually quite a bit more to it. Traditionally, a person who has found their *ikigai* has found something to do with their life that meets the following four criteria:

1. Something you love

2. Something you're good at

3. Something the world needs

4. Something you can make money from

I have a patient who is forty-three years old and a writer. He lives with his wife and two dogs and they have chosen not to have children. He spends his days writing. He loves it, he's quite good at it, he writes insightful pieces that make the world a better place and he makes money from it. His whole life is about his writing. Even when he's walking the dogs, he's thinking about his work, dictating thoughts and ideas into an app on his phone. How many of us are this lucky? Not many, for sure. How many of us could radically reorganize our lives and families so that we could live this way? Even fewer. Achieving *ikigai*, as defined by these four criteria, is a huge ask.

It would have been an even lovelier story if Simon could have somehow found a way to make a living by opening a shop for collectors in the high street and quit his job. But just because he hasn't achieved all four aspects of *ikigai*, that doesn't mean he hasn't made progress. He's discovered his passion, his mission, his joy. Sadly, many of us aren't even trying to achieve this. It does appear, however, that this is starting to change. Millennials and Gen-Xers are developing a reputation for seeking out professions based upon a sense of purpose and an active desire to do good in the world. Many of them say that doing something they're passionate about is a long-term goal. The twentieth and early-twenty-first centuries have brought us many benefits, but so much of it has been material. We're only just beginning to grasp the fact that *things* don't make us happy. They're a drain. It's what we *do* that truly changes the texture and structure of our lives.

L.I.V.E.

Unless you're very young and are lucky enough to have the resources and opportunities to enable you to pursue your passion in such a way that it becomes your job, achieving *ikigai*, as judged by the above criteria, is probably an unrealistic goal. This is why I've taken the core insights from this wonderful philosophy, combined it with everything I've learned over nearly two decades of helping my patients heal and thrive and formulated my own progressive solution. I call it L.I.V.E. and it has four core elements:

LOVE. INTENTION. VISION. ENGAGEMENT.

L.I.V.E.

LOVE. INTENTION. VISION. ENGAGEMENT.

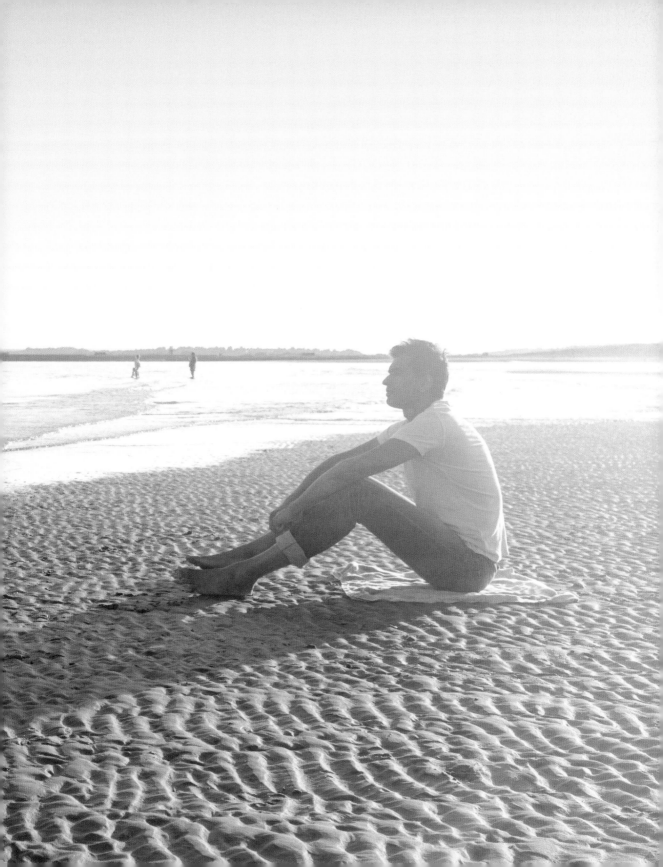

L.I.V.E.

The first involves doing something you love, the second is about living with intent, the third is developing and working towards a long-term vision, and the final one is about engaging with the world around you. I'm not expecting you to find just one pursuit that manages to cover all four elements.

It's completely OK to try to hit each one through different pursuits and activities in your life. You may not be able to hit each one immediately, either – that is fine. Take Simon, for example. When I first met him he was disillusioned and stressed out with his job. When I suggested that he do something he loved, he started playing with his train set, which gave him his lust for life back. Interestingly, he came in to see me just a few weeks ago about something completely unrelated and told me how much more enjoyment and fulfilment he is now getting from his job. By doing something that he loved, it nourished him on the inside. This then allowed him to reframe and reflect on his job in a different way. He was now able to see that his job was an opportunity to engage with others in wider society, as well as fulfilling the important role of feeding his family. When he had no passion in his life, he couldn't see this.

Every aspect of the L.I.V.E. framework is connected. Once you get started, I believe you're likely to find that your life becomes brimming with meaning and purpose. You'll be happier, calmer, less reactive and, perhaps most crucially, way more resilient in the face of those inescapable daily MSDs. I don't know of a better way of transforming your life, and yourself, than this.

LOVE: DO SOMETHING YOU LOVE

A few years ago I found myself going through a very dark time. I was caring for my sick father and working long hours in a stressful, busy practice. During that period I had a brief respite on a stag do up in Edinburgh. That weekend I happened to meet someone who lived just around the corner from me. He told me he used to play a lot of golf in his teenage days but hadn't picked up his clubs in over a decade. I'd always been curious about the sport but hadn't played much myself. After a couple of pints, we made a pact that we'd get together as soon as we could and start to play regularly.

When I got home and looked at my diary I realized that the only way I could honour my promise was to arrive at the course at 6.15 on Saturday mornings and play for just two hours. But what a difference it made. As I got more and more into it, I started to notice that, no matter how stressful my week had been, everything felt better in the days that followed the game. I'd be less reactive to the MSDs that were flying at me because I'd given myself a bit of meaning-nourishment and allowed my emotional brain to switch off. In the downtime of my commute, instead of ruminating, I'd be picturing the green, the slopes and all the techniques that I was determined to master during our next session. I'd spend every spare minute reading golf magazines, practising my swing in the mirror or visualizing the course. Golf books piled up beside my bed. I'd wake up thinking about my new passion.

This first element of L.I.V.E. is to do with your reason for getting up in the morning. It doesn't have to be your job. It doesn't have to be your children. As important as career and family undoubtedly are, often our thoughts about them are too enmeshed with our responsibilities towards them. This is about something that brings joy and feeds you internally which you want to do for intrinsic pleasure rather than to gain social media likes. Preferably, it's also something you can get in touch with every single day, even if it's spending twenty minutes on an internet forum with friendly, like-minded people or sitting down with paper and pencil, planning exactly what you're going to do when you next get the opportunity to throw a few hours at it.

I want you to find something that you're thinking about doing because you want to do it, not because you *need* to. Don't worry if finding out what it is takes a while and you try a few pastimes that hold promise but, ultimately, don't set you on fire. Discovering what we *don't* like is part of the process of realizing what we *do* like. And try not to post about it on social media. You'll find the joy and pleasure stay with you for longer if you make this just about you.

If you pursue potential new passions without judging yourself in the process, you may well discover that what brings you true joy is something creative. It could be painting, dancing, drawing, playing a musical instrument, singing, knitting or even sculpting. Society teaches us that some people are 'creative types' but, actually, we're all naturally creative. The problem is that the adult world, with all its anxieties and responsibilities, stifles it. I wholeheartedly agree with the legendary painter and sculptor Pablo Picasso, who once said, 'Every child is an artist. The problem is how to remain an artist when you grow up.' Modern life tries to make us into consumers rather than creators. I often reflect on the balance between these two opposing forces. I'm convinced that the underlying cause of so much of our stress these days is the constant pressure to consume more than we create.

One clue that you've found the thing you love is that time, and even your sense of self, will seem to vanish when you're busy with it. Psychologists call this 'flow state'. It encourages the growth of your rational brain because, when you're fully immersed in something, it's extremely difficult for your emotional brain to take over and trigger a whirlpool of negative thoughts. Kids, when they're completely taken up with the games they're playing, are a great example of being in flow. The distinguished psychologist Mihaly Csikszentmihalyi, who originally coined the term, believed that you can only really achieve flow when you're challenged. His work showed that, when we're in flow, we experience less stress.

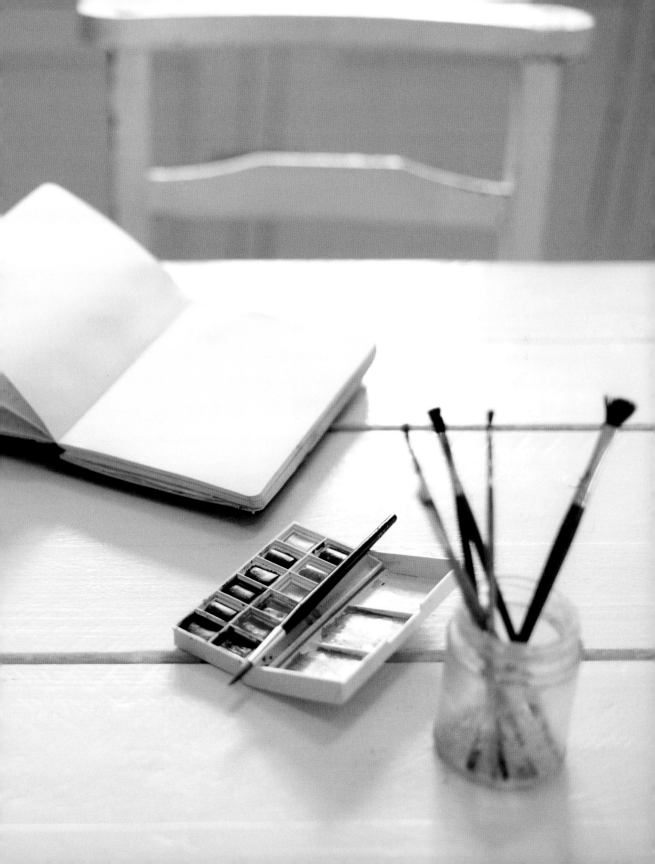

INTENTION: DO SOMETHING WITH INTENT

Most of us live day to day without much thought, on the never-ending treadmill of life, putting one foot robotically in front of the other. This second element to L.I.V.E. is all about trying to break out of that trance at least once a day. It's about being more attentive and learning to take pleasure in the small things. Consider what happens when we do something as simple as making a cup of tea. We flick the switch on the kettle, drop a tea bag into a mug and wait impatiently until the kettle boils, then splash a bit of milk in and get out of there.

Compare that to the Japanese, who have complex rituals that have evolved around the making of tea. While I realize that modern Japanese people aren't ritualizing every cup of tea they make, and I'm not expecting you to follow these ancient rites in practice, I would like you to mimic them in spirit.

I want you to do something each day, no matter how small, with real mindful intent. Examples might include cooking a meal without distraction, or having a shower while being mindful of the warm water flowing down your body, or brushing your teeth while paying full attention to the sensation you feel on each and every tooth, or making a cup of tea while mindfully watching the steam rise as you slowly pour water into the cup. I believe that when we start paying attention to the small things, the big things start looking after themselves.

In the years leading up to his death, my father began a daily intent practice almost accidentally. Throughout his entire life, he'd never shown any interest in domestic pets. But when he was stuck at home, unable to work or do much else, the neighbour's cat would often come and sit on our drive to bask in the sun. One day Dad gave him a bowl of milk and the cat quickly got used to this and would come for his treat. Dad began to look forward to this simple pleasure. Some days, he'd be up early, waiting by the door, looking out for the cat. Even though his vision was failing, he was frail and he couldn't move around much, he'd always hobble to the fridge and pour out the milk. He'd often spill some of it on the kitchen floor, but that didn't matter. The broad smile on his face triggered by this simple, intent-ful act was a joy to witness. I'm convinced it's little things like this that helped him cope with being chained to a hospital haemodialysis machine three times a week, for so long.

VISION: DEVELOP A LONG-TERM VISION

While intent is about meaning and purpose on the day-to-day level, this third element of the L.I.V.E framework is to do with the long-term roadmap of your life. In his classic book *Man's Search for Meaning*, Viktor Frankl, an Austrian psychiatrist who survived the horrors of Auschwitz, writes powerfully about the critical importance of having a long-term goal. 'Everyone has his own specific vocation or mission in life; everyone must carry out a concrete assignment that demands fulfilment,' he wrote. For Frankl, the difference between those who survived and those who didn't was that sense of purpose and that long-term goal. He focused on what he needed to do, which was complete his manuscript, and lived.

Your brain is smarter than you probably realize. It's always planning ahead. If you have a specific and clear long-term vision, it will always be helping you get there. It's easy to underestimate how important this is. When we know the 'why' of our lives, we automatically reduce our stress load. Research indicates that we're able to endure short-term struggles with much more resilience if they're helping us achieve our long-term goals.

I'd like you to write down a goal that you would like to achieve over the next twelve months. Think about what you want and the steps you'll need to take to achieve it. And then, most importantly of all, take that first step. You have to take action, no matter how small it is.

ENGAGEMENT: DO SOMETHING THAT MAKES YOU ENGAGE WITH OTHERS

When she was thirty-six years old a patient of mine, Amanda, quit her hectic job in sales in order to raise her first child. Three years later, she gave birth to a second child. This baby, a daughter called Billie, had trouble feeding and soon developed behavioural problems. This meant that Amanda was fully caught up in dramas of everyday life as a mother for seven or eight years, until Billie was old enough to attend school. Suddenly Amanda found she had spare time. But rather than this being the start of the new, more chilled-out and happier period in her life she'd long imagined, she started bickering with her husband. Before she knew it, she was battling psychological problems which I was worried might potentially develop into an eating disorder.

When I talked to her in my surgery it seemed clear that Amanda was missing a very big something. She told me she didn't know who she was any more. I spoke to her about potential creative pursuits she might enjoy, but nothing seemed to grab her. Then, one day at the school drop-off she met another mother who was looking for someone to help her with her fledgling online business. She was after someone who could proofread copy that would go online. Amanda volunteered. It was only two or three hours a week, and it didn't pay anything more than a weekly batch of home-made flapjacks, but soon everything started to change. Amanda felt wanted and useful and that she was doing something meaningful for someone else, someone who really needed her help. Interestingly, her attitude to her home life quickly improved too. It became apparent that a lot of the angst she'd experienced at home with her partner was coming from a deep dissatisfaction with other parts of her life.

I believe the thing Amanda needed so badly was engagement. True fulfilment is so often in the giving. Humans are social animals and we are often at our happiest when we're acting in the service of others.

I'd like you to do at least one thing every day for someone else. And no cheating – I mean something *extra* that you don't *have* to do. It could be making a cup of tea for a new colleague in the office, saying hello to the cashier in the supermarket and asking how they are, picking up some litter in the street or holding a door open for someone. These small acts of kindness will boost your self-esteem and help infuse your daily life with purpose. As time goes on, you'll begin to significantly reframe your sense of self as you come to view your existence as profoundly valuable. If this final core element gives you the buzz I think it will, you might consider taking up some voluntary work.

LEARN TO L.I.V.E. TO LIVE

If everything is information, then the best thing you can tell your body and brain is that your days are useful and rich and that, despite inevitable hiccups and difficulties, you are thriving. Without any purpose or meaning in your life, you can end up being blown about like leaves, buffeted by life's endless MSDs. If you practise the 3 Habits of Calm (affirmations, reframing and gratitude), schedule your time and begin working with the L.I.V.E. framework (love, intention, vision and engagement), I believe you will start to live a life that's profoundly less stressful. Finding your purpose isn't about adopting some grand project. It's not about changing the world, becoming a millionaire entrepreneur or writing a bestselling novel. It's simply about making a bit of space in your day to nourish the thing that most needs looking after and which you've probably been neglecting for too many years: you.

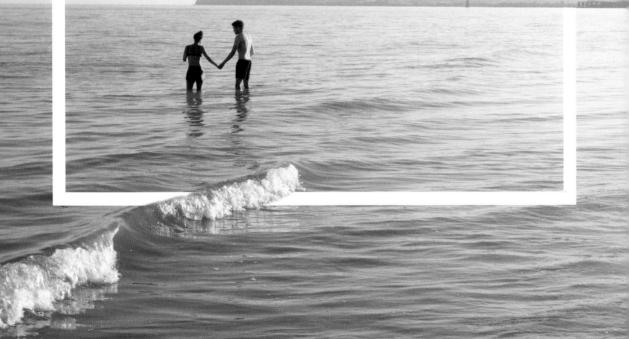

2/RELATIONSHIPS

We're all living ultra-connected lives. In our pockets we have tiny technological miracles through which we can communicate, instantly, with anyone on the planet. We're blessed to have such amazing power at our fingertips. We've never been so connected to the rest of the human race. At least, this is what we're constantly told. But I don't buy it. The nutritional equivalent of the kind of connection we're having today is a can of fizzy pop and a chocolate bar for breakfast. It's industrialized, transactional and inhuman. So many of the stress-related problems I see in my surgery have as a root cause a chronic lack of connection. This lack of connection is a major stressor in our lives and is having a devastating effect on many of our relationships.

But nourishing relationships can also help us destress. We feel happy when we are connected to friends, family and those around us. Social constructs have evolved to facilitate and improve the way we live as a community, but now 'social' media has exploded. As a result, we are no longer feeling connected in the same ways and are more isolated than ever before. We need more 'social' and less 'media'.

In this pillar, we will explore three distinct areas that I have found, over the years, to be major sources of twenty-first-century stress: a lack of human touch, the insidious erosion of intimacy and the deprioritization of friendship. In each section, I will give you actionable strategies that will improve the quality of your relationships, from simple ways to nourish your brain with more human touch, to one of my personal favourites, the 3D greeting!

Chapter 4
HUMAN TOUCH

As a young GP I used to really struggle when I had to give someone bad news. When there was a diagnosis of cancer, say, the thing that helped most of all was sitting close to the patient and putting my hand on their arm or shoulder. That small gesture was a comfort to me and, far more importantly, to the person I was speaking to. The sad thing is, we're living in a world that's becoming averse to touch. While there are reasons for this, I'm beginning to worry that we've gone too far. These days, I'm extremely nervous about making even the slightest physical contact in my clinic. Simple touch is now seen as crossing a personal boundary. I understand why this has become the norm, but have we lost something vitally important in the process?

Humans are mammals, and touch is part of our deepest mammalian systems. It is the very first sense we develop as a foetus. Being touched as a child helps form vital neural pathways and feeds emotional connections. A lack of touch can have devastating consequences. Up until the 1990s, appalling orphanages existed in Romania in which the children were fed and watered but grew up without experiencing any touch at all. They were later studied by psychologists, who found that almost all of them had developed serious behavioural problems. As adults, they had difficulties attaching to others and some even suffered delayed development of the gut. Interestingly, the children who had even the briefest moments of affectionate touch from volunteers didn't suffer these problems to the same degree.

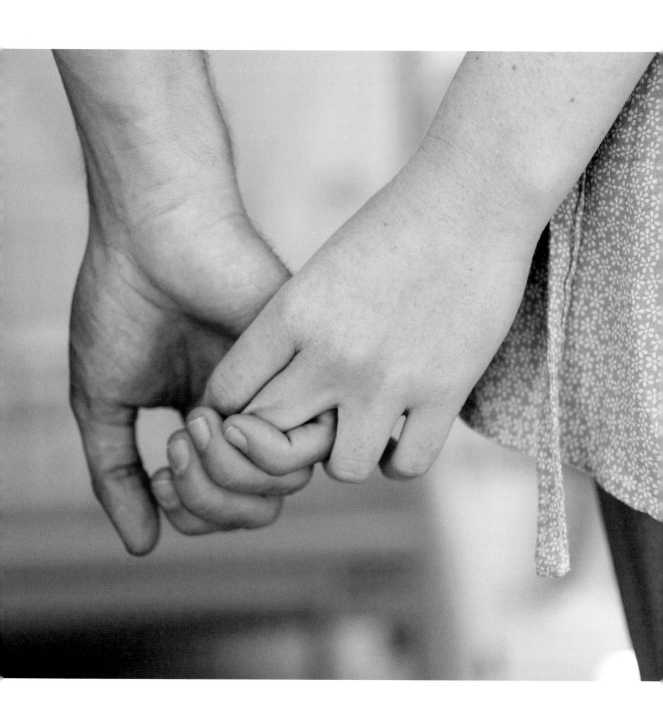

Studies on rats have found that pups whose mothers lick them a lot grow up to be relatively calm. These pups have cortisol receptors that are more sensitive, which means they can better regulate their response to stressful experiences. In contrast, pups whose mothers don't lick them enough grow up to be hyper-responsive to stress. If these pups were humans, they'd be the kind of person for whom every little thing is a stressor. They'd always be looking at the negative and would have a generally pessimistic and anxious outlook.

Studies on humans confirm the primal importance of physical touch. Members of basketball teams who use more hands-on interactions with each other perform better, ending up higher in their leagues. If a waiter taps you on the shoulder as they give you a bill, you'll be likely to tip more. When people visiting a library were treated in a tactile way, they reported a much more positive experience than those who weren't touched. Researchers at University College London found that affectionate touch reduces feelings of social exclusion, which is one of the most painful experiences a human can have. That study's lead author, Mariana von Mohr, wrote, 'As our social world is becoming increasingly visual and digital, it's easy to forget the power of touch in human relations.' Human touch can slow down our heart rate, lower blood pressure and reduce our cortisol levels. It even raises the levels of Natural Killer (NK) cells. NK cells are part of our body's innate immune system – that is, the hard-wired branch of our immune system that we are born with. They are a key part of our armoury to fight off threats, such as infections and cancer cells.

And, even beyond the data, we know how good we feel when we get a hug. You feel a warm sensation rushing through you. The skin is giving information that things are going well in our social world. Without touch, we're not accessing this rich network of systems that evolution has put there for a specific purpose. One of the world's top researchers in touch, Professor Francis McGlone at Liverpool John Moores University, has said that touch is 'not just a sentimental human indulgence, it's a biological necessity'. A lack of touch is a physical stressor on the body and helps throw you into a stress state.

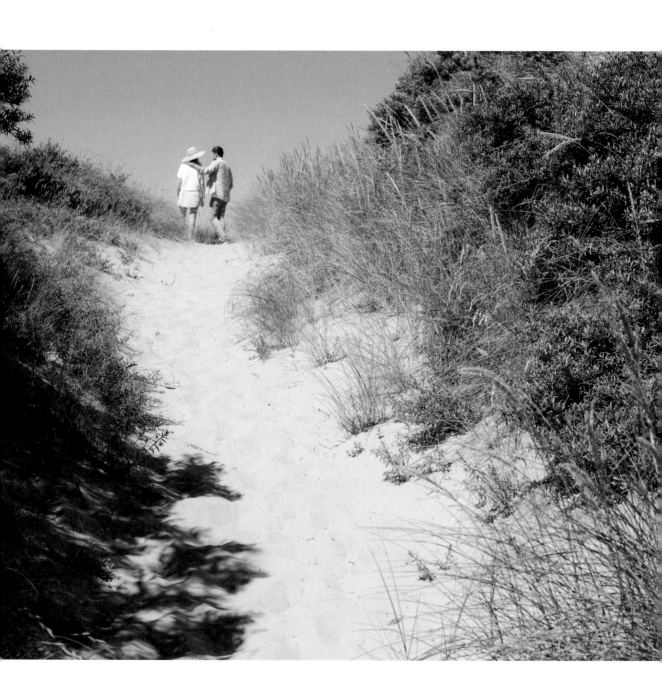

GET IN TOUCH WITH HUMAN TOUCH

Amazingly, there's still much we don't know about the workings of affectionate touch in the body. We do know, however, that it has functional similarities to pain. Humans have two different types of pain nerve fibres: fast and slow. The fast nerve fibres give us basic anatomical information, simply letting us know where exactly the pain is so that we can take immediate remedial action. The second type of nerve fibre is the slower one. This gives the pain its emotional quality.

You'll probably recognize the two different pain responses if you think about what happens when you grab a hot pan. Firstly, you have an immediate form of pain that tells you it's too hot and causes you to drop it. That's the fast pathway. A few seconds later, the second, slower pathway kicks in. This is the emotional component – you feel shocked, upset, you might wail or even cry. I recognize this two-step process whenever I see my daughter fall over. Initially, she's a bit bemused by what's happened and might put her hand on the area that's been hurt. But a few seconds later, when the 'emotional' quality of the pain has reached her brain, she starts to cry.

This same two-step process occurs with touch. There is a fast nerve fibre that simply lets us know where we've been touched, giving us the physical sensation. But there's also a slow nerve fibre system that feeds our brain on a much deeper level. These slow nerve fibres go to one of the most primitive systems in our brain, the limbic system, which helps mediate our emotions. This system is what gives touch its deep, nourishing quality and is especially triggered by stroking.

THE STROKES

Back in December 2017 I was lucky enough to visit Professor McGlone's lab as part of a BBC documentary series I was filming. I was blown away by what I found. These slow nerve fibres are called the C-tactile (CT) afferents. These CT afferents take the touch signal from the skin to the limbic system, deep within the brain. They respond to a specific kind of light, stroking touch that occurs at a speed of roughly five centimetres per second. Any faster or slower, and these nerve fibres become less responsive.

If you ask someone to stroke a wooden arm, the pace and the depth of their stroke will be all over the place. But if you ask that same person to stroke a human arm, they *automatically* lock into a stroke whose speed is approximately five centimetres per second. It turns out this is exactly the same speed that people rate as most pleasant. This shows how deeply embedded affectionate touch is in our biological and neurological systems. It's not learned, it's primal. Mothers intuitively caress their babies in this way.

This is why applying cream or moisturizer to the skin can be so soothing. It's also why, when infants are stroked at that particular speed, their heart rate decreases. The CT afferents are connected directly to the hypothalamic–pituitary–adrenal (HPA) axis, which acts as our stress broadcast service (see p. 16). When we're stressed, it broadcasts a series of messages throughout the body which ultimately put it in a stress state. McGlone is finding that, simply by stroking the skin, we can directly soothe the HPA axis and lower our cortisol levels. Pleasant, affective touch also directly lowers our stress levels by increasing the tone of the parasympathetic nervous system, which puts us into a thrive state.

The Benefits of Affectionate Human Touch

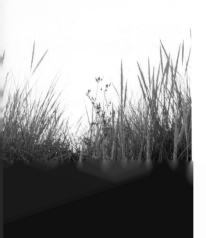

Lower heart rate

Lower blood pressure

Reduced cortisol levels

Raised levels of Natural Killer cells (one of the immune system's defences against infection)

Increase in parasympathetic tone, which puts us into thrive state

However, it is important to remember that not everyone appreciates being touched. We all have our own experiences and cultures that shape the way we interact with each other. It is important to respect others' personal space – an unwanted touch, however innocent, can be perceived as threatening by another person.

REWARD PATHWAYS

Professor McGlone also told me about a touch version of a well-known study called the Marshmallow Test, which is used by psychologists to judge willpower in children. Youngsters are offered a sweet treat and are told they can have it right away or wait for a certain amount of time and have a larger portion. The test is famous because it's been shown that the longer children are able to wait – the more willpower they show – the better their lives tend to turn out in the long run, in terms of health, happiness and wealth. In this version, the person offering the child the treat touches them on the shoulder. When the child is touched like this they're able to defer the reward for longer, when compared to a control group. McGlone speculates that this is because, with that simple touch, the children have had their internal reward systems topped up.

What's really interesting about this is that we have a particularly high concentration of these specialized touch receptors on our back and on our shoulders, which is exactly where the children had this brief moment of human contact. It's remarkable that we have so many of these receptors on areas of the body that we struggle to access easily ourselves. These touch receptors give us pleasure and by being present on hard-to-reach areas, they would have promoted behaviours that would have ensured that those body parts got touched. Evolution must have placed them there so we could receive touch from other people.

But for these receptors to have stayed on our back and shoulders through millions of years of evolution, there must also have been a benefit for the giver of touch. Indeed, we know that those who give affectionate, gentle touch are rewarded with increased levels of endogenous opioids, compounds made by the body that act on opiate receptors and are associated with improved mood, decreased pain and lower anxiety. These are the same effects we get from exogenous opioids such as morphine. I find it incredible that evolution has gone to such lengths to promote us being with others, and it is hard to make the case that we have evolved to be anything other than social beings. This is the theme running throughout the Relationships pillar – we are designed to live and exist with others. The quality of our relationships is key, and touch plays a critical role.

Although this chapter is primarily focused on human touch, these touch-giver benefits are well known to those with pets. Although not a pet owner myself, I have spoken to many patients and friends who tell me that when they are feeling stressed they spend time stroking their pet and their stress levels immediately plummet.

McGlone believes a lack of touch from others could be at the root of some of society's biggest problems. He feels that if the brain does not get appropriate nourishment from pathways that have been honed over 3 million years of evolution, it will crave that nourishment elsewhere. This could be a contributing factor behind rising levels of addictive behaviour, such as the misuse of drugs and alcohol, and gambling. McGlone also believes that touch could help reduce the stress schoolchildren experience when taking exams. He's started investigating whether increasing peer-to-peer touch helps buffer them from the effects of stress and cortisol induced by examination pressure.

You can listen to a detailed conversation between Professor McGlone and myself on my *Feel Better, Live More* podcast at drchatterjee.com/touch.

THE TOUCH TRADE

One of the reasons touch feels good is that it triggers the release of serotonin, commonly known as the 'feel-good chemical'. Many antidepressant drugs work by trying to increase serotonin. The recreational drug ecstasy acts on the serotonergic pathways and is one of the reasons why ecstasy users have a heightened sense of touch and find touch more rewarding when under the drug's influence. Touch can also change levels of the so-called 'cuddle chemical', oxytocin (see p. 112), as well as endogenous opioids (see p. 91).

Given that touch is so essential, and feels so good, it's hardly surprising that an industry is growing up around it, with professional 'cuddlers' and 'touch' workshops increasingly available. Massage therapy is also becoming incredibly popular. There are many types of massage, and they differ in force and velocity. However, all of them are known to have benefits on the way that we feel and on our stress levels. Light-touch massage probably stimulates the CT afferent nerve fibres, and there's evidence that it stimulates the release of oxytocin too. High-force massage such as Thai massage is thought to release endogenous opioids.

HEALING TOUCH

Just by coincidence, in the weeks leading up to my meeting with Professor McGlone, my seven-year-old son had started saying, 'Daddy, stroke me,' as I was tucking him into bed. I wondered where this had come from. I now know that my son was craving that deep and powerful CT afferents response. Since then, I try to ensure that I spend a bit more time every evening stroking both my children on their upper back or arm. I've come to believe that the touch I give my children is just as important as the food that goes into their bodies and the physical activity they do.

It also gave me a new idea of how to help a tricky patient, Ivy, who I'd been seeing for over a year. She'd come in with a thyroid problem and I'd been helping her change her lifestyle. Ivy would frequently contact my surgery. If even the smallest thing went wrong, she was desperate to get hold of me instantly. She was single and told me she always seemed to attract men who were in relationships already and only interested in seeing her on the side. I felt that I'd done as much with her physical wellbeing as I could, so I started exploring her emotional world. It turned out that Ivy was never touched as a child. Her parents never showed her love, either verbally or by stroking her. As a child, she always craved affection. Her environment was giving her the information that she wasn't good enough, and that's what she came to believe. It occurred to me that this lack of physical nourishment was a significant Macro Stress Dose and perhaps at least partly responsible for her constant worrying. She had some close girlfriends who she saw regularly. 'When you see them,' I asked, 'do you hug them?' She bristled at that. It was as if I were suggesting something revolting. As an experiment, I asked her to start hugging them. A few months later she told me she felt much warmer towards her friends and she'd even started forcing herself to hug her mother. While this turned out not to be a solution to her wider problems, I suspect it significantly raised her personal stress threshold, because I'm no longer getting as many panicked phone calls as I was.

KEEP A TOUCH DIARY

Touch nourishes our body in crucial ways, much like food does. Just as you need to eat every day, you need human touch every day. And remember, there are benefits for the giver as well as for the receiver.

I'd like you to keep a touch diary to discover just how many times you give and receive gentle, warm, affectionate human touch. Tally your total by the end of the first week. By the end of week two, double it. Then, by the end of the month, triple it.

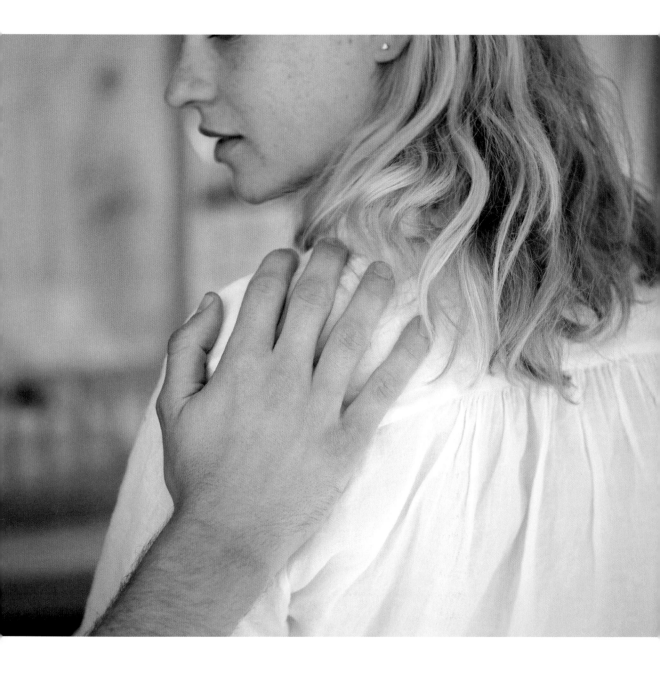

SIX WAYS TO GET MORE TOUCH

1. **Hug someone close to you each day,** if possible – family, friends, even work colleagues.

2. **If you have children, make an effort to hug them at every opportunity.** This is important whatever their age – not only for babies or young children, but also for older children, above the age of ten.

3. **If you have an elderly friend or parent,** try to ensure some level of physical touch whenever you see them, such as a prolonged warm embrace.

4. **Try roughhousing with your kids –** play-fighting involves a lot of human touch and it's thought that this kind of play helps children develop emotional resilience. You can do this with adults as well!

5. **Book a massage.**

6. **Give someone a pat on the back when giving them praise.**

Chapter 5
GET INTIMATE

Reni and Saul were not having sex and it was damaging their marriage. Despite being only in their mid-thirties, they found themselves feeling increasingly distant, emotionally and physically, from each other, and this was making them bicker. They both worked for the same tech company, putting in long hours, usually into the weekends. Reni was looking for a quick-fix solution. 'How does Viagra work?' she asked. Her husband glanced at her reproachfully.

'Well, before we think about that, have you tried scheduling?' I said.

'What, scheduling *sex*?' asked Reni, clearly horrified.

'It doesn't have to be sex,' I said. 'It could be just lying naked in bed together, showering together, even taking a nap together. Set some time aside for it once or twice a week.'

She paled and shook her head, muttering, 'This feels like a business arrangement.'

'You don't think scheduling is romantic?' I asked, to the sound of Reni's barely stifled laughter.

What I told Reni and Saul next seemed to shock them. I find the idea of romance deeply problematic. Romance is what teenagers do, and those in the first blushes of their relationship, when they can't keep their hands off each other. It's courting behaviour, but it's behaviours we've been conditioned by our culture to expect to last for ever. This just doesn't happen. The romantic model, which is fed by pop music, Hollywood and fiction, has given us an impossibly high bar to meet, especially in the hectic world we live in today, in which both partners in a couple will often work and may have young children or adolescents to look after.

Research tells us that we are having less sex now than we have for decades. Americans are having 15 per cent less than in the 1990s and, in the UK, rates have fallen by over 20 per cent in under fifteen years. This rate of decline is alarming.

Rather than expecting romance, I believe that adults should instead focus on intimacy. Intimacy doesn't have to come with fireworks, vintage champagne and roaring log fires. It doesn't even have to be sexual. But if you don't actively schedule it – in between the school run and the emails from the gas company saying you're six weeks late on your meter reading – it won't happen. So I asked Reni and Saul to park their scepticism and give it a go. Two months later, they were like a different couple. And the irony was, by throwing out any expectation of romance, they found that was exactly what came back into their marriage.

THE MODERN WAR ON LOVE

Modern life asks too much of love relationships. Many of us already feel overburdened, with adult couples having to shoulder the responsibilities that a whole village would once have shared. In previous times, members of the community would have given emotional nourishment and support but today, all too often, we live miles away from our friends and family and expect our partner to share our financial and emotional responsibilities. And on top of all that, we expect them to be a sexual partner too.

Because so much practical load is put on our relationships, they can become seriously malnourished. Many of the couples I see tell me that the only time they can work on their relationship and spend valuable time together is on 'date night', which, as often as not, is cancelled at the last minute when other, more 'important', things come up. Needless to say, technology isn't helping. I used to relish long car journeys with my wife, especially in the evening. The kids would fall asleep in the back, and we'd chat. Over the past few years, though, things have started to change. I started to notice that Vidh would spend a lot of time on her phone, surfing the net or texting her friends, while I was driving. This didn't really appear to be a problem at first but, bit by bit, I noticed that the atmosphere in the car had started to change – the intimacy was simply not there.

When I brought the topic up with my wife, initially it didn't go down so well. You see, I probably brought it up in an accusatory fashion and Vidh probably felt defensive and in denial. A few weeks later, however, we managed to have a calm and productive conversation about it and decided to try to implement a new rule. Barring emergencies, we were going to try to be off our phones on long car journeys together. Instead, we would prioritize this as time for ourselves, when we had none of the distractions that would so often suck up our time when we were at home – such as the washing-up, the housework or preparing the kids' lunches. Since we made this change, our long car journeys have been completely transformed. They are now filled with meaningful and deep conversation – the intimacy has returned.

ENDING THE iAFFAIR

Reni and Saul also had problems that stemmed from their use of tech. It became apparent, as I talked to them, that they were addicted to their smartphones. Once upon a time we worried about our partners having an affair with a work colleague, but these days we're all having extramarital relationships with our devices. Our phones are the last thing we think about before going to sleep and the first thing we think about when we wake in the morning. It's our phone that we can't keep our hands off, whose every curvy contour we know by touch and whose buttons we know exactly how to press to turn them on. It's our phones we're thinking about during romantic meals and our phones we really want to be with when we're lying in bed with our spouses. Our phone is the third member in our relationship.

This is an affair that just has to end if we're finding the intimacy is draining from our relationships. Fifteen years ago, in the evening a couple would talk over dinner, then they might have the shared experience of watching television. At bedtime, there would have been dim lights and communication and cuddling that would, at times, lead further. But it's extremely common now for partners to go to bed and be on their devices. This keeps them siloed in their own digital worlds. Even as they sit centimetres away from each other, they might as well be on either side of the planet.

With the advent of on-demand TV and streaming services such as Netflix, couples are frequently going to bed at different times, with one staying up late to binge on a boxset. There is nothing inherently wrong with bingeing your way through multiple episodes of *Homeland*, but if this is coming at the expense of meaningful connection time with your partner, there will be a knock-on effect which will show up in other areas: more bickering, perceived problems in the relationship and a lack of intimacy.

In my surgery, I'm seeing a lot more people coming in complaining of a lack of libido – more than I ever have before, in nearly twenty years of seeing patients. One of the dangers is that this lack of an urge to have sex is often interpreted as a sign that something is badly wrong in the relationship. This is yet another serious stress to have to bear and, more often than not, it's actually untrue.

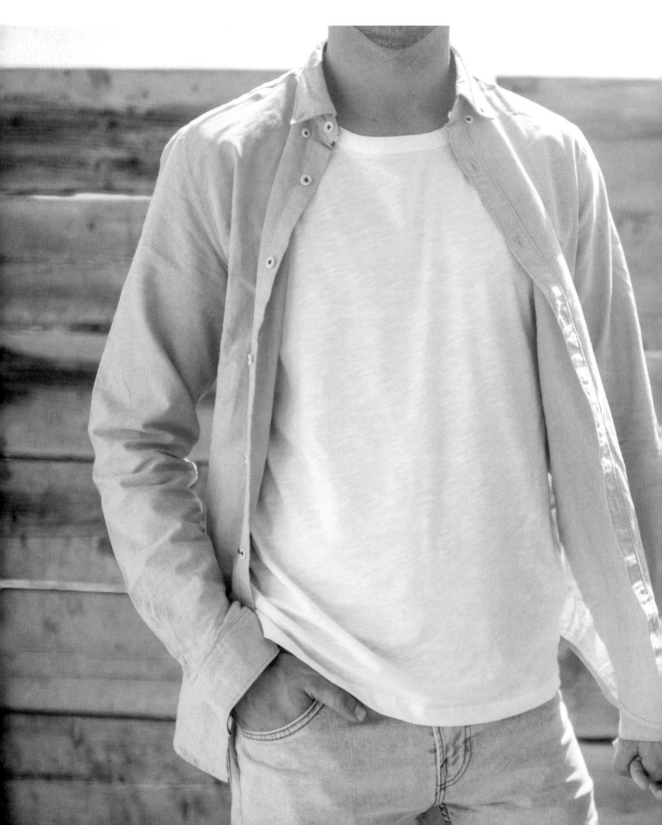

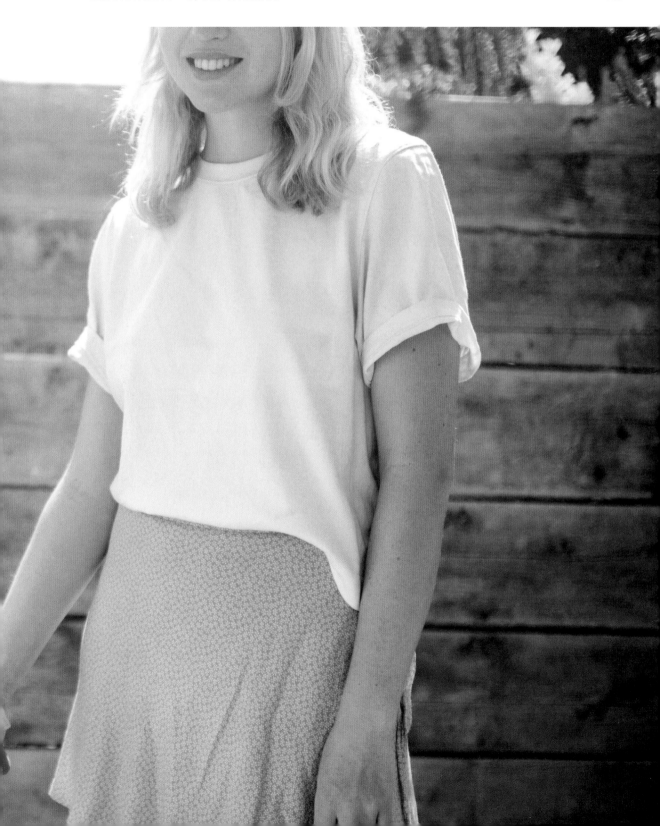

WE DON'T HAVE TO TAKE OUR CLOTHES OFF

Intimacy doesn't necessarily mean sex. From conversations with my patients, I would say it has several components:

1. Trust

2. Feeling like two members of a team

3. Being responsive to each other's needs

4. Being present with each other

5. A deep level of care for the other person

6. Sharing profound information – thoughts, desires and wishes – with each other that you would not share with anyone else

As you can see, sex does not feature on this list. Sex can occur in an intimate or non-intimate way and is not in itself a requirement for intimacy. Just holding hands with your partner can be incredibly intimate. In fact, studies show that when a woman is holding her husband's hand, she reacts better to stressful events. Although this study was done on women, I have no reason to believe that this effect is sex-specific.

Similarly, if somebody takes a shower or a nap with their partner, it also has benefits. Even something as simple as sustained eye contact can be transformative. I experienced this last year when I met a meditation teacher who made a lecture hall full of doctors do an exercise which I have to confess was one of the most uncomfortable I've ever experienced. We were all randomly assigned a partner and asked to sit opposite them with our knees touching and our eyes closed. We then had to open our eyes and stare into the other person's for five minutes.

It was as unforgettable as it was uncomfortable. There were times when it became so intense that either my partner or I would have to look away. But I soon started to pick up things about my partner's character and what they were feeling. At the end of the five minutes, even though we'd not said a single word to each other, I felt as if I had formed a deep connection with this person, to the extent that, as my partner was a woman and I'm a married man, I thought it might border on being too much of a connection. Then it occurred to me that I didn't think I'd ever done anything like that with my wife. So I went home that night and we tried it. Those minutes of sustained eye contact had a powerful positive effect on the texture of our relationship that remained for days.

SEEING EYE TO EYE

I would highly recommend that you try this exercise with your partner or a close friend.

- Sit opposite your partner or friend, ensuring that your chairs are close enough so that your knees are touching.

- Close your eyes for between twenty and thirty seconds and concentrate on the sensation of your knees touching.

- Now open your eyes and look directly into each other's eyes.

- Try to maintain eye contact for a full five minutes. You may need to set a timer on your phone or have a clock to hand.

- If you do find yourself looking away, gently reinitiate eye contact as soon as you can.

- After the five minutes is up, take some time to share your experience with each other. How did it feel? What went through your mind? What did you pick up about each other during that time?

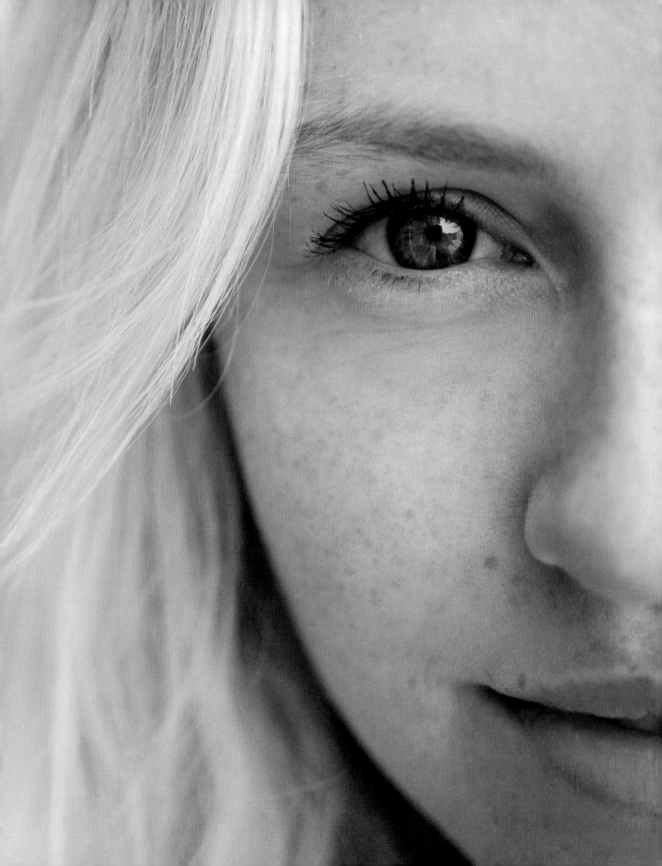

THE 3D GREETING

All this got me thinking. So many of us are 'too busy' for this kind of simple intimacy. Familiarity, in a love relationship, all too often breeds complacency. You've been working from home on your computer all day, your partner walks in and you barely lift your head up from the screen. Or you've just come back from a long day at work and you walk in, yet your partner barely says anything. It's heartbreaking, almost literally, how the daily grind makes us treat our husbands, wives and long-term partners.

In the months after I married Vidh I was working in Oldham, very near my wife's parents' house. Once a week, I'd nip over to have lunch. Vidh's dad also worked nearby and would also pop home for lunch. I'd notice that whenever he arrived her mum would drop everything, go to the door and greet him with a smile, eye contact and a kind word. Sometimes she'd touch his arm or place her hand on his shoulder. It seemed a little old-fashioned at the time, but now I'm convinced they were on to something.

Those small, loving moments I saw back in Oldham and that powerful eye-contact exercise inspired me to start greeting Vidh in a new way. When I see her in the morning, I now greet her in three dimensions – with eyes, touch and voice. Giving my wife a heartfelt 3D greeting makes all the difference to our day. The way I feel in myself is different – less stressed and more supported in my relationship. The effect is still lingering when I see her again that evening; there's just a bit more closeness than there would be if we were just like passing ships, and talking only about the management of the following day: who's picking up the kids? Who's going to the supermarket? And it takes less than fifteen seconds. We're all busy, but I've never met anyone who's so busy they can't spare the love of their life fifteen seconds. Try greeting your loved ones in this way and see for yourself.

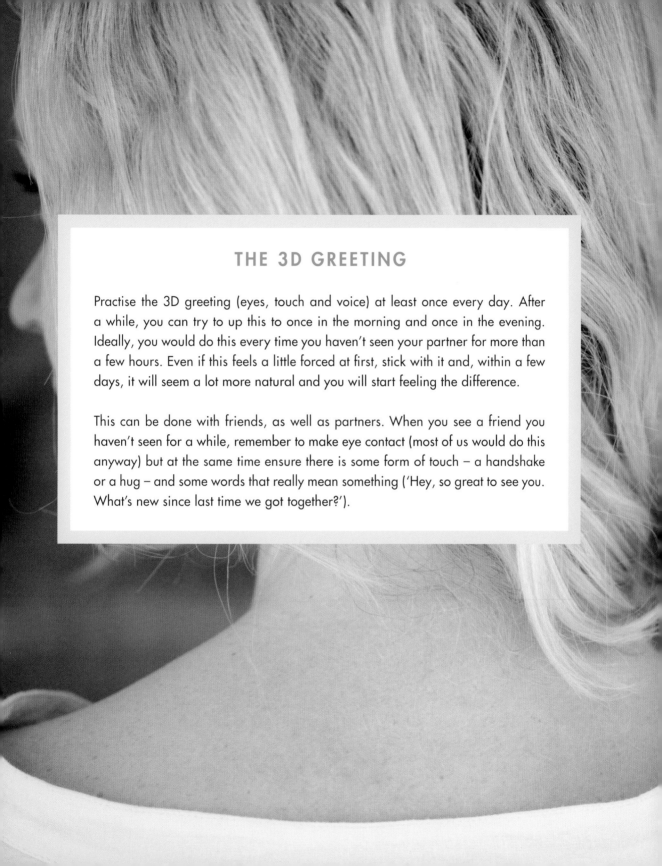

THE 3D GREETING

Practise the 3D greeting (eyes, touch and voice) at least once every day. After a while, you can try to up this to once in the morning and once in the evening. Ideally, you would do this every time you haven't seen your partner for more than a few hours. Even if this feels a little forced at first, stick with it and, within a few days, it will seem a lot more natural and you will start feeling the difference.

This can be done with friends, as well as partners. When you see a friend you haven't seen for a while, remember to make eye contact (most of us would do this anyway) but at the same time ensure there is some form of touch – a handshake or a hug – and some words that really mean something ('Hey, so great to see you. What's new since last time we got together?').

TESTOSTERONE

It's unfortunate for long-term relationships generally that the human libido can be so fragile. When we feel tired, our libido goes down. When we feel busy and stressed, our libido goes down. One of the main reasons is because modern living is affecting our levels of testosterone, which in turn can affect our libido.

People often associate testosterone with masculinity and strength and, while it is crucial for men, it's also important for women. Low levels of testosterone in women have been associated with low mood as well as muscle weakness and fatigue.

When we're stressed, the body prioritizes the production of cortisol over the sex hormones, such as testosterone. This makes perfect sense evolutionarily: if we're in danger, our body is going to put its resources into survival rather than procreation. Twenty-first-century living sends our body signals that we are under threat. We are no longer running away from the dinofelis; we are being attacked by our modern lives. This is becoming a big problem for the Western world. Overall, an astonishing 40 per cent of the US population is low in testosterone.

Potential benefits of increased testosterone:

Improved bone strength	Increased cognitive function
Improved libido	Improved body composition
Increased lean muscle mass	Better overall drive for life
Increased strength	

SEVEN WAYS TO INCREASE TESTOSTERONE

1. **Get more sleep.** A lack of sleep causes ageing in both men and women. One study found that men who sleep only five to six hours per night have testosterone levels equivalent to men ten years their senior.

2. **Minimize stress as much as possible.** When we're stressed, the body prioritizes cortisol production over testosterone production. The recommendations throughout *The Stress Solution* will help you.

3. **Resistance training is excellent for increasing testosterone.** You don't need a gym to do this: bodyweight exercises or my five-minute kitchen workout from *The 4 Pillar Plan* are easy ways to get started.

4. **Aim to eat a minimally processed wholefood diet.** This will help with hormone production.

5. **Minimize your alcohol intake.** Increased alcohol intake is associated with lower testosterone levels. It is a good idea to stay within government guidelines and drink less than fourteen units per week.

6. **Maintain a healthy body weight.** As belly fat increases, the activity of an enzyme called aromatase goes up, which converts testosterone in your fat cells to oestrogen.

7. **Limit your exposure to Bisphenol-A (BPA).** BPA is a synthetic chemical found in many plastics. Studies have linked BPA exposure to lower testosterone levels. A recent study reported that 89 per cent of men attending a fertility clinic had BPA in their urine.

THE MAGIC OF OXYTOCIN

The benefits of intimacy are likely mediated by a hormone called oxytocin. Sometimes known as the 'cuddle chemical', oxytocin also functions as a neurotransmitter, which means it helps nerve cells communicate with each other. It's produced in a part of the brain called the hypothalamus. From there, it's transported to our pituitary gland, where it's released into the body's bloodstream, through which it exerts some of its pleasing effects.

While calling it the 'cuddle chemical' is rather simplistic, it does have some truth to it. It helps the uterus to contract during childbirth and is involved with the secretion of a mother's breast milk. It's also implicated in the experience of orgasm and research has shown us that it's involved in empathy, trust and social connection. When we bond socially with someone, our oxytocin levels go up. In addition, it's thought to be crucial in the maintenance of long-term relationships. When a couple have sex, the afterglow of warm feelings they feel for each other is partially the effect of all the oxytocin they have washing through their systems. And animal studies have shown that the presence of oxytocin seems to buffer us from the effects of stress, partly because it reduces the amount of cortisol that's released.

MAKE A PLAN FOR INTIMACY

Everything in life is easier when we have a sense of intimacy running along in the background. It's the glue that holds relationships together. We're often too busy for intimacy, and I see the consequences of this in my practice every single day. By having a plan to create more of it, you'll find that your stress levels go down and your resilience goes up.

FIVE WAYS TO NURTURE INTIMACY
WITH A LOVED ONE

1. **Schedule regular time to connect and be intimate without the distraction of technology.** Date nights may be a bit of a cliché but they are a fantastic way to prioritize intimacy. It could even be a commitment to spending thirty minutes with each other every evening without your smartphones in sight, or simply a daily walk holding hands.

2. **Give your partner a massage.** If this feels a little bit intimidating, you could start off by holding hands or massaging cream on to their feet or arms.

3. **Steal intimate moments together whenever you have the time.** Always look for opportunities in your daily life to be intimate and present with each other.

4. **Smile when your partner walks in through the door, even if you don't feel like it.** As I mentioned on p. 64, our actions will very often determine our mood. This action means that intimacy will become the norm rather than the exception.

5. **Remember the 3D greeting (eyes, touch and voice) at least once per day.** Make deep, meaningful eye contact, embrace warmly and exchange a few loving words.

Chapter 6
NURTURE YOUR FRIENDSHIPS

Humans are not designed to be alone. We've evolved to live our lives as individual members of a large, supportive group. Back when the human brain was doing much of its evolution, we hunted together, we ate together and we sat around a campfire in the evenings and talked together, swapping stories, songs and smiles. We raised our children in sprawling extended families, an invaluable network through which the relentless workload having kids brings was dispersed. Those same extended families cared for their elderly, giving them sustenance, both nutritionally and socially.

But this is not how we live today. Modern parents typically juggle intense work pressures with looking after kids and find themselves with less and less time even to talk to their friends, let alone gather with them every day to unwind, laugh and de-stress. Our elderly folk end up in care homes, staring out of windows for hours at a time, or at daytime television. A rising number of us are suffering from loneliness, and it's not just the elderly. A recent study by the Mental Health Foundation found that eighteen- to thirty-four-year-olds were more likely to feel lonely than those over fifty-five. Scientists have long known how toxic social isolation can be. As far back as 1979 it was found that people with the fewest social ties were three times more likely to die prematurely than those with the most. Being lonely means you're 30 per cent more likely to have a stroke or a heart attack. In fact, high social stress is an even bigger risk factor for dying from a chronic disease than physical inactivity, alcohol intake and smoking – put together.

While it's obvious how loneliness can make us feel unwell mentally, it's less clear how it can have such an impact on our physical health. But the fact is that loneliness, like so much else that affects our wellbeing, is information. Because we've evolved to live as a single cell in the larger organism of a mutually supportive human tribe, when we feel isolated the brain reacts as if something's wrong. It thinks we're in danger. Back when we were hunter-gatherers, being isolated from the tribe would have been a death sentence. Loneliness is telling the brain: 'I don't have my tribe around me. I'm not safe. I might not be able to feed myself. I no longer have access to the tribe's places of shelter. If I come under attack or injure myself, I'm in mortal trouble.'

When the brain and body feel like they're in a place of danger, there is only a limited menu of options of how to prime the body to deal with it, and one of the favourite go-tos is inflammation (more on this in 'De-stress Your Diet' on p. 134). George Slavich, a researcher at the University of California, Los Angeles, found that rejection and isolation switches your genes into a more inflammatory state. Over the long term, this makes your immune system weaker and predisposes you to a variety of life-threatening conditions, including type 2 diabetes, depression and obesity.

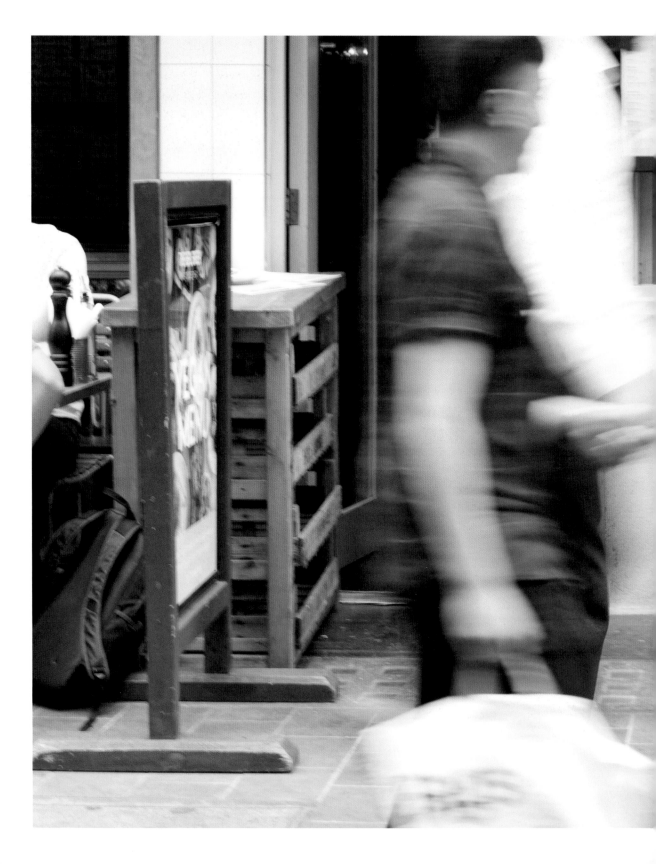

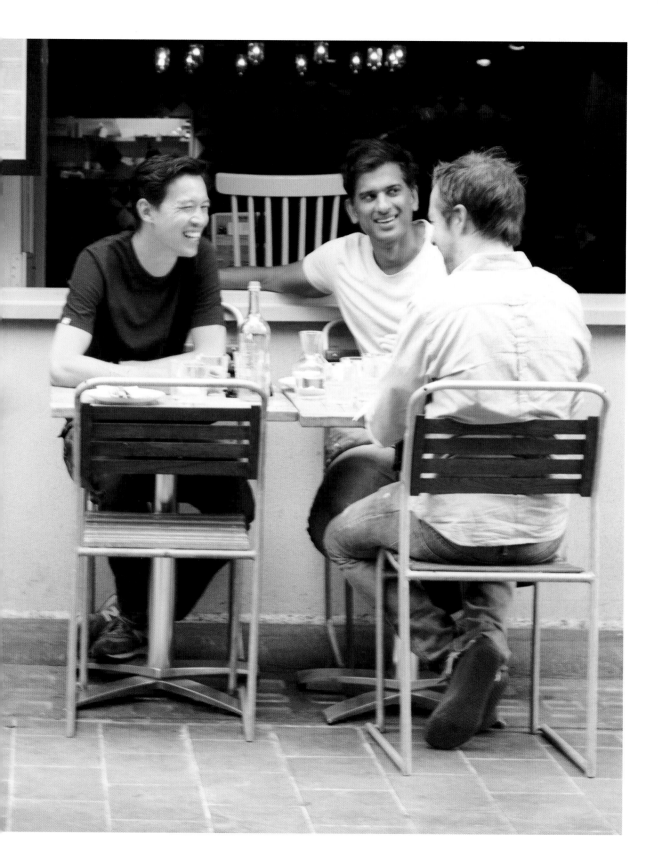

PUBS AND CHURCHES

There are a whole variety of reasons behind the current epidemic of loneliness, and many of them have to do with major changes in how we work and play as a nation. Up until very recent times pub life was stitched into the fabric of the existence of millions of Britons. Yes, people went there to drink alcohol, but for most pub-goers that wasn't the pub's only purpose. It was a place to get together, to share stories and experiences and to discuss any issues that were worrying you. It was the twentieth-century equivalent of the tribe's campfire. The local church would have fulfilled the same role. But the first two decades of this millennium have seen huge declines in the numbers of pubs and churches in the UK. I believe these changes have been an enormous source of national stress, but nobody seems to be talking about it.

Although we certainly don't have the same café culture as France or Italy, I have noticed that people are now starting to get at least some of what they've been missing from pubs and churches over cups of tea and coffee. A few years ago, I got into the habit of stopping at a local café on the way to my surgery at 6 a.m. and ordering a black Americano. Morning after morning, I'd sit with my drink and savour it. Soon I began to recognize all the regular faces. We'd chat about what we'd been up to, discuss our plans for the day and talk about what was going on at home. On one occasion, my boiler had broken down and, instead of jumping on the internet and trying to find a plumber, I asked at the café. That got me thinking that this was like a local community. We evolved in groups in which we protected one another, pooled resources and worked together. This was exactly what was happening there. I was getting the same kind of value and interaction that people used to get from tribes, pubs and churches.

BECOME A REGULAR

Whether it's going to your local café at the same time every day for a coffee, or going to a club, church or recreation centre, regular visits somewhere and a happy, open demeanour should lead you to becoming connected to a new group of people. Some examples include:

A weekly yoga or Pilates class

Participate (or even volunteer) in a weekly Parkrun

Join a local sports club – table tennis, snooker, cricket, badminton or a martial art

Join a local walking club

Volunteer to help a local group, such as the Cubs or the Guides

Have Sunday lunches with your neighbours

Join a local book club

Get involved with the rapidly expanding cycling community

Take a regular class or workshop in a passion you wish to pursue, such as painting, sculpting, writing or learning a new language

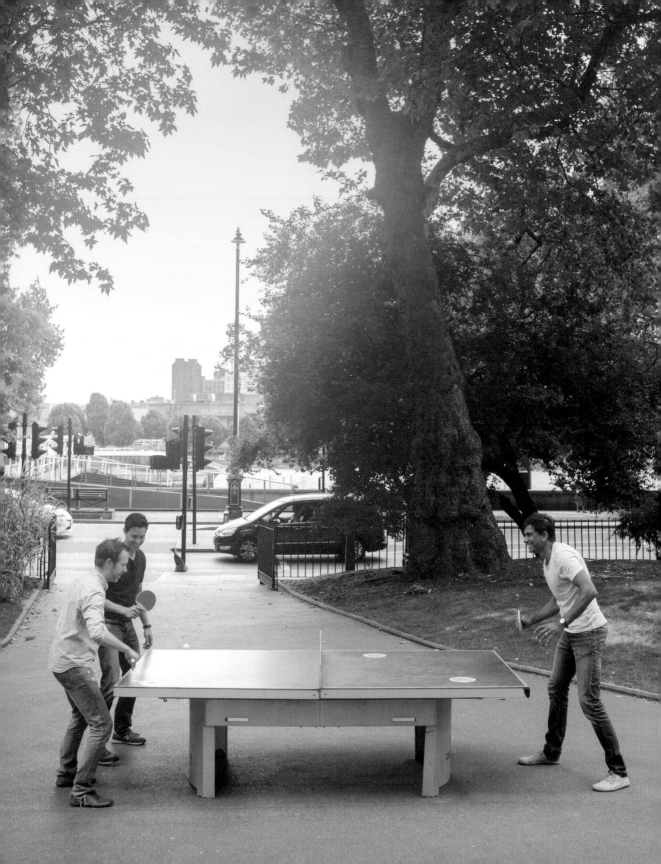

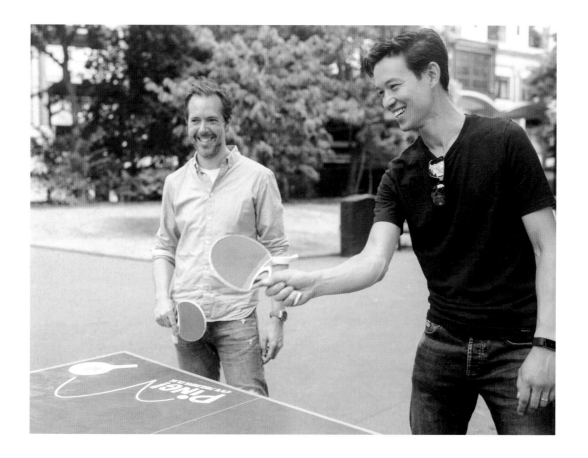

FAKE FRIENDS, FAKE COMMUNITIES

Of course, one way we're plugging the gaping hole that's been left by the decline of our community institutions is by making connections on social media. But Facebook friends are not always 'real' friends. Likes and comments are no substitute for hugs and conversation. Even the way we interact online is different. One poll of 2,000 people found that roughly 25 per cent of them admitted making personal remarks to others online they'd never say if they were standing in front of them in real life. The revolutionary psychologist Professor Robin Dunbar, who specializes in research into our tribal, evolutionary history, has said that 'People are more prone to saying something on social media that they later regret, because in these digital environments, we don't receive the immediate checks and balances that we get during normal face-to-face interactions.' When we're on the other end of these negative comments, our bodies react as if we're under attack. These are responses that have been hard-wired into our DNA over millions of years, switching on when we feel socially isolated and rejected.

Another problem with online communities is that they change the way we get our sense of self-esteem. Everyone's feelings of worth are tied, in part, to their sense of status. We all desire status, and Professor Mitch Prinstein from the University of North Carolina has written about the two very different forms it comes in: popularity and likeability. Facebook or Instagram 'likes' focus us on popularity, which encourages narcissistic, me-focused behaviour. This is a stress on the body, quite literally. If you feel disappointed when a post you make doesn't gain any traction, that's a form of rejection, and it will impact you on a genetic level. It's information, to your brain and your body, that you're not bonding with your 'tribe', which will flip you into a stress state.

While social media can be wonderful if you use it to connect with people who share your interests and learn from those you admire, it's important to be aware of the dangerous lure of popularity. Instead, try to prioritize likeability, which is the healthier form of status and is associated with much better life outcomes. It's other-focused, not me-focused, and makes us concentrate not on how much we're impressing our peers but on how likeable they find us.

Personally, I don't really call someone a friend until I've met them. A recent study estimates that it takes about fifty hours of time spent with someone to make a 'casual friend', ninety hours for them to move up to the status of 'friend' and two hundred hours before you can consider someone a 'close friend'. This makes a lot of sense to me. Many of my closest friends are from my university days, when you get to spend hours and hours together. The fact is, people you're interacting with online can only ever be peripheral to your life. You can't truly know someone unless you've breathed the same air as them.

MAKE *MOAI* MATES

Thousands of miles away, in Okinawa, Japan, you can find the people who live longest in the world. The Okinawans have a concept of *moai*, groups of five friends who have committed to each other for life. Not only is this a wonderful idea, it's also telling us something valuable about friendship. Feeling connected is not about the number of friends you have but about the quality of those friendships. If something really exciting is happening in my life, there're only a few people I want to jump on the phone to share it with. It's the same when something bad happens that I want to talk about. These are my *moai* mates.

But with our busy lifestyles it's often hard to keep such friendships nourished. Not only are we busier than ever but perhaps we feel we don't need to catch up with our mates so much. After all, we 'know' what they are up to – we've seen their holiday snaps, photos of their kids, where they ate last weekend on our social media feeds. I find it remarkable that on your birthday you can receive between fifty and two hundred messages wishing you 'Happy Birthday'. Of course, it is great to receive these messages, but is it really the same as one of your close friends remembering your birthday and actually making a call?

Loneliness is on the rise these days. In fact, it is such a problem that the UK government has recently appointed a Minister for Loneliness. Although it can affect everyone, it does seem to be an issue that is disproportionately affecting men. Men are four times more likely than women to commit suicide and, on average, currently eighty-four men a month are committing suicide in the UK. While there are many factors that contribute to this, it is clear that the lack of a close group of friends is a significant contributor. In fact, the rate of male suicide has been linked to a steep drop-off in friendships after the age of thirty. Two and a half million men in the UK are reported to have no friends at all with whom they could discuss a serious topic such as worries about work, health, family or money. Women tend to find it more socially acceptable to spend time together – meeting up with a 'girlfriend' to go for a drink, a trip to the shops or a weekly fitness class, for example. Many men don't feel as if they can do that.

With pubs and other places for regular meet-ups gradually disappearing and the change in societal roles, many men feel a sense of isolation. In my practice, when I see men like this, we discuss ways in which they might be able to spend some time with people who share a similar outlook. Sports clubs can be great for those that way inclined, but see also the suggestions on p. 119. There will almost always be an option for everyone.

DIARIZE TIME WITH YOUR FRIENDS

Make sure that you are regularly diarizing time to meet up with your friends, in person. The frequency will depend on many things including workload, family and distance. For my university friends and I, who all live hundreds of miles away from each other, twice a year for a few days is what we can realistically manage. If you live near to your friends, perhaps every two weeks or once a month will work fine.

Meeting up with your friends is not a luxury, it is an absolute necessity for good health. Why not pick up the phone right now and call your friends to arrange a get-together – what are you waiting for?

THE CONNECTION PRESCRIPTION

THERE IS NO MAGIC NUMBER. Don't feel you need to have five *moai* mates. You may have one. However many you have, try to have one interaction every week with someone that goes to the heart. If you don't feel that you have even one, try some of the strategies in the box on p. 119 to start meeting some people who share your interests.

PLANNING MAKES MATES. At the start of the year, think about your *moai* mates. Who are they? Have you got face-to-face meet-ups penned into your diary? My closest friends live hundreds of miles away from me, but I try to arrange to meet them at least twice a year. If your friends live locally, can you meet them once a week?

CONFESS YOUR STRESS. I have a friend who was raised a Catholic. Although he's no longer religious, he remembers how powerful the experience of confession was and how elevated and relieved he felt when he left the church having told an anonymous priest about the chocolate biscuits he'd stolen from the cupboard. I believe that Catholics have developed a powerful comfort instinct (see p. 25) in confession, and it's one that we can replicate in our *moai* interactions. We could begin by being unafraid to confess our stress. We shouldn't be ashamed of the fact that we're struggling. We shouldn't feel we need to keep a stiff upper lip at all times. Stress doesn't mean you're a failure, it means you're human.

HAVE RISKY, MASKLESS CONVERSATIONS. I love what Gandhi said: 'True happiness is when what you think, what you say and what you do are the same thing.' This is what I strive for, although I'm certainly not there yet. We spend most of our lives trying to project an image to others. Whether we're at the school gate or at work or having dinner with our parents-in-law, it's very rare that we can let that mask down. *Moai* mates are ones with whom you can let your guard down, be authentic and take risks in what you say and do, secure in the knowledge that they get you and will always have your back.

'*True happiness is when what you think, what you say and what you do are the same thing*' – Gandhi

WRITE LETTERS. I find that communications online are usually transactional rather than meaningful. We exchange information, but it's rarely an exchange that nourishes us. My parents were born and raised in India and I still have vivid memories as a child of blue airmail envelopes arriving in the post. Mum would be so excited. With trembling fingers, she'd open the letter, stop everything and spend five minutes reading it from beginning to end. Her parents would have written the letter three weeks previously. Back then, international phone calls were extremely expensive and not that reliable. For my mother to phone her parents, she'd have to call a local operator, who'd then try to put her through to a local phone box, and even then the chances of getting hold of her parents were very slim. So these airmail letters had real value. The whole letter told a story: you could get a sense of the smell of India in the house; you got something from the ink that was used, and the handwriting, some of which was squeezed in at the tops and the sides just so it could all fit on the page. There's something so precious and intimate about letter-writing. It takes thought and care and, when your handwritten letter arrives at its destination, it'll be a precious moment for the receiver.

MOVE ON WITH THANKS. Don't be afraid to move on from friends who no longer nourish you, who don't allow you to be yourself, who don't want to hear your innermost thoughts or support you in your most vulnerable moments. This sounds harsh, but it's crucially important. You don't need to do it with animosity or regret. You can be grateful for the time you've spent with them and the purpose they served at the time. Don't feel guilty about it. Life moves on. People change. Your drinking buddies from college may not be the people you choose to spend time with today. That's OK.

3 / BODY

We feel stress in the body. When we're having a bad day and those Micro Stress Doses (MSDs) are flying at us, we experience them as physical sensations: the tightening in the shoulder; the lurch in the stomach; the dryness in the mouth; the restless motion in the leg. These are the immediate bodily reactions to stress. But what's not so intuitively obvious is that the body can also be a *cause* of stress. Just as your brain constantly monitors your environment for information, assessing whether you're in a threatening place or not, it also monitors your body. If the signals sent from the body are bad, we become stressed. This pillar's going to tell you how you can change the information that your body is emitting. By making a few simple decisions about how you eat, move and organize your day, you can start living much more of your life in a healthy, happy thrive state.

Chapter 7
EAT YOURSELF HAPPY

Over the past few years I've been through a personal revolution in my understanding of how important the things we choose to eat are to our psychological wellbeing. This crystallized for me back in 2015 when I read an editorial in one of the most prestigious medical journals in the world, *The Lancet*. The editorial claimed that 'nutrition may be as important to mental health as it is to cardiology, endocrinology and gastroenterology'. This was a simply amazing claim. Could it really be true that our food choices affect the functioning of our minds to the same extent that they affect the health of our hearts and stomachs?

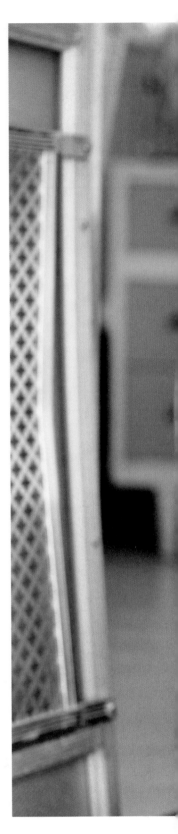

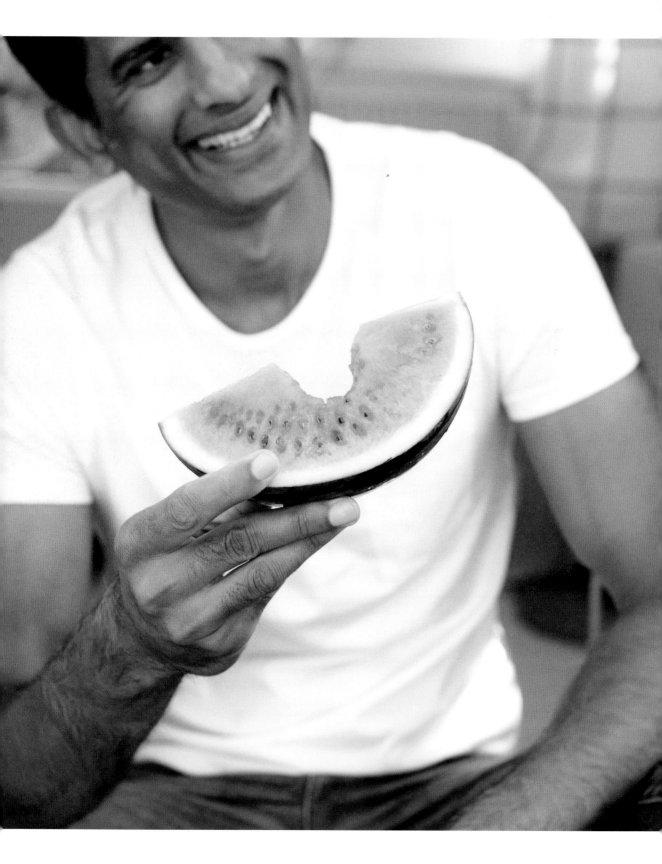

It just so happened that, at the same time, I was treating a patient in my surgery who'd been suffering with an especially tricky set of mental health issues. There was no mystery as to the initial cause of forty-eight-year-old Biba's problems: she'd been in a horribly traumatic motorway accident in her early twenties and had experienced bouts of extreme anxiety and panic attacks ever since. She felt stressed from the moment she woke up until the minute she went to sleep. She'd seen countless doctors and had tried a whole range of antidepressants, none of which really helped her. She'd also been referred to counsellors, but she found the impact of talking about the crash too painful and kept disengaging.

I quickly realized that Biba had developed a number of coping mechanisms that centred on her food choices. She'd buy meal deals from a high-street shop and would eat a lot of highly processed food throughout the day: sugary cereals, chewy lollies, biscuits and sausage rolls. 'Yes, there are serious emotional issues that we need to tackle,' I told her. 'There's no question about that. But you've already tried going down that route and without much success. I think we should change tactics and take a look at your diet.' She was a bit resistant at first, and I completely understood why. Her problem was psychological. How on earth could the living nightmare she'd witnessed on that motorway be counteracted by a piece of steamed haddock?

But after prolonged discussion I convinced her to try. I helped her come up with five simple meals that she'd enjoy – natural, minimally processed food with a wide variety of colourful vegetables. With the support of her family, she started to cook fresh every day at home. Six weeks later I discovered that the change had been utterly remarkable. Her mood had become more stable and her daily anxiety attacks had reduced by around 70 per cent. All this simply by changing what she put into her mouth.

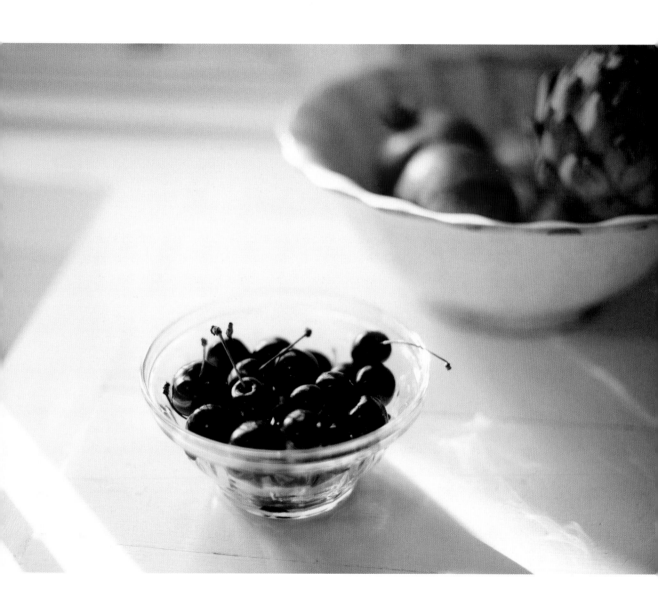

DE-STRESS YOUR DIET

Before we get too carried away, this is not a story of miraculous reversal. Biba's problems didn't vanish completely. Rather, this is a story about stress being a feed-forward cycle. Biba's trauma had triggered changes in her body which made her crave highly processed food. This food threw her body into stress state and this stress state amplified her mental health problems further, which caused yet more changes in her body, and so the spiral went around and around. My intervention was enough to break that cycle. After a couple of months Biba realized she was able to cope emotionally with the psychotherapy she'd previously found so hard. Ultimately, her life was transformed, and it all started with her diet.

Seeing the change in Biba and reading about all the new research that's been coming out on the links between nutrition and stress have led me to completely rethink my previous assumptions. And not a moment too soon. According to the mental health charity Mind, one in four of us is going to experience a mental health problem in any given year. And yet at a recent lecture in Bristol I asked over a hundred GPs, 'How many of you discuss food with patients who complain of stress and anxiety?' and was disappointed to see only about 5 per cent of them put their hands up. There is an urgent need for medical training to catch up with the latest advances in scientific research.

The response I got at the lecture was also a product of how reductionist our cultural thinking around food usually is. When we look at our meals, we need to start asking ourselves, 'Is this going to give my brain the information it needs to thrive? Or is it going to make it think it's under attack and cause the body to throw its defences up?' This is the choice we make every time we put something in our mouths.

HOW FOOD BECOMES INFORMATION

We're used to thinking of food simply as fuel. It goes in one end, the body breaks it down, the protein goes to our muscles, the carbohydrate gives us energy, the fat goes to our thighs, bum and belly, then all the stuff it doesn't want is deposited out the other end. We're not used to thinking of that cheese-and-pickle baguette as something akin to a radio station or a book. But, effectively, that's what it is. The body reads information from that baguette then sends it to the brain. The nature of that information is the result of a three-way interaction between your food, the bugs that live in your gut and your immune system. Whenever you eat, those three systems talk to each other. The conclusion of all that complex biological chatter is then sent to the brain. It's information, telling it whether or not the body is under attack from bad food.

THE GUT–BRAIN AXIS

When we talk about having a 'gut feeling' about something, we reveal that we've always intuitively known that there's a direct line of communication between the digestive system and the brain. There are in fact several communication super-highways between them and, collectively, they're known as the gut–brain axis. Research is ongoing in this area but so far we know that some of the information flows from the gut to the brain via the lymphatic system and some of it travels via little messenger cells called cytokines that are made in the gut and travel to the brain through the blood. Some, however, is sent directly to the brain via the longest nerve in the body, the vagus nerve.

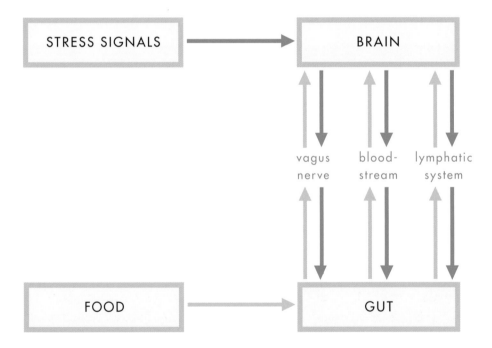

WHAT HAPPENS IN VAGUS

The vagus nerve is one of the most important highways in the gut–brain axis. It emerges from a part of the brainstem called the medulla oblongata, a region that plays a crucial role in automatic functions such as breathing and sneezing. From there it takes a long and winding route to get down into the gut. And it's bi-directional, which means it carries information from the brain down to the gut, but also from the gut back up to the brain.

A key part of that information stream comes from an incredible and mysterious world that we didn't have much understanding of until recently. Your gut is inhabited by massive populations of different bugs – bacteria, viruses, fungi, parasites and their respective genetic material – that, in total, weigh about as much as the human brain. This hidden world is our gut microbiome.

These bugs interact with the body, with the food we eat and with each other. These interactions determine many aspects of our health and mental wellbeing. As amazing as it sounds, if we treat these microscopic organisms poorly, they can make us feel anxious and depressed. If we treat them well, they can lighten our mood.

Studies on animals find that an absence of gut bugs increases our reactivity to stress. This has led to some scientists calling them 'our brain's peacekeepers'. Keep them happy and they keep the peace. So, how do we keep our gut bugs happy? By cutting out the highly processed and refined foods that damage them and feeding them with food that nourishes them. This includes colourful plant-derived wholefoods rich in fibre such as vegetables, fruits, legumes and pulses. Feasting on these kinds of foods means they can make highly valuable compounds such as short-chain fatty acids (SCFAs) that can communicate with the brain. These SCFAs can travel directly to the brain via the bloodstream. But they can also send signals via the vagus nerve. They send flashes of information to the brain telling it that everything is OK.

YOUR INNER FOOD TESTER

But it's not only your gut bugs and your brain that are involved in this constant conversation about whether you're safe or in danger. Your immune system is also involved in the chatter.

Part of the immune system's job is to sample every single thing we eat, checking whether it's OK or potentially harmful. If we eat bad food, it responds by triggering a process called inflammation.

This is one of our basic and ancient evolved responses to stress. It puts our bodies in a state of heightened alert, ready to fend off anything foreign and unwanted that might invade our systems as the result of an injury such as a bite from a predator, say, or a dirty cut.

Humans are designed to experience inflammation in short, sharp doses. As we learned earlier, having it over a longer period of time – what's known as chronic inflammation – can be extremely bad for us. Chronic inflammation is at the heart of many serious complaints that I see in my surgery every single day, whether it is insulin resistance, type 2 diabetes, obesity, high blood pressure or depression.

The food that we eat, our gut microbiome and our immune system are intimately linked. The right kind of food promotes a healthy microbiome, which in turn helps to train and educate the immune system, making it much more likely to produce a critical type of cells called 'regulatory T-cells'. These cells help to dial down the immune-system response, reducing inflammation in the first place and keeping us out of stress state and firmly locked in thrive.

LEAKY GUT

Another way that diet can throw us into stress state is by causing what's colloquially known as 'leaky gut'. This happens when poor lifestyle and food choices damage the integrity of a very delicate but critical barrier that sits between the gut and the rest of the body, making it too permeable. This increased permeability allows harmful substances from inside the gut to slip through and gain access to our bloodstream.

Among the worst of these substances are lipopolysaccharides (LPSs), which sit on the outer coat of certain gut bugs. If the LPSs stay inside your gut, all is fine. But you really don't want this stuff in your blood. If you were to inject LPSs directly into your veins, your body would start to shut down and you'd enter septic shock. Of course, when you develop a leaky gut you don't suffer such instantaneous effects. It's much more insidious than that. Every day your gut will leak tiny amounts of LPSs into your blood and that will put your immune system on high alert, causing inflammation and pushing your body out of thrive state and into stress state. We know that LPSs can contribute to a number of different health problems including depression, low mood and anxiety.

THE MODERN WORLD'S ASSAULT ON OUR GUTS

Most of your gut bugs live in the depths of your large intestine, but rather than it being a safe, damp cave system for them to securely thrive in, your bugs are actually very vulnerable down there. Modern life, it seems, is at war with our bugs. Highly processed foods, such as ready meals, biscuits, many breakfast cereals and some highly processed breads, can have a terrible effect on their health. Some additives, emulsifiers, pesticides and artificial sweeteners can decimate them as well as antibiotics used in food production. When this happens, stressful signals will flash up to the brain via the vagus nerve and other pathways in the gut–brain axis. This is yet another mechanism by which poor nutrition can trigger us to feel psychologically unwell.

Popular drugs, including heartburn medications and antibiotics, can have a similar annihilating effect. While some people's microbiomes are able to recover from a course of antibiotics in about a week, others seem to be far less robust. Some can take two years or more to recover, if at all. As a GP, when I'm looking at the history of patients who are struggling with their mental health and anxiety, I now take a detailed history of how many antibiotics they've used.

I'm seeing more and more of a correlation between those who have high anxiety or problems with stress and those who have had a huge intake of antibiotics, particularly as a child. I try to go as far back as I can into their medical history. Even being born via Caesarean section can lead to potential problems – incredibly, most of our microbiome is seeded when we travel through our mother's vaginal canal.

THINGS THAT CAN DAMAGE THE MICROBIOME

- Eating highly processed food

- Drinking too much alcohol

- Smoking

- Drinking sugary soft drinks

- A lack of diversity in your diet

- Overuse of antibiotics and other medications

- Psychological stress

- Over-exercising

- Lack of sleep

- C-section birth

- Living in urban environments

- Hyper-cleanliness and the use of too many antibacterials

- Eating foods containing emulsifiers (chemicals that are added to lots of highly processed foods, to keep the texture consistent)

- Artificial sweeteners – animal studies have shown that they can be detrimental to our gut microbes. While more research takes place, I urge caution.

If several of these apply to you, please don't worry. In the twenty-first century, pretty much all of us will have experienced at least one, if not many more, of these attacks on our microbiome. We can't change the past, but we can make positive changes to improve our gut health in the future. Following the recommendations in this chapter will help you feed and repair your microbiome, and growing evidence suggests that high-quality probiotics can be a helpful adjunct for some.

THE SCIENCE OF EATING HAPPY

Scientific studies are only just beginning to reveal the powerful link between food and our mental wellbeing. In 2017 a gold-standard randomized controlled test known as the SMILES trial put patients with severe depression who were already undergoing treatment on a modified Mediterranean diet of oily fish, colourful fruit and vegetables and wholegrains. Twelve weeks later these patients had a much greater reduction in depressive symptoms than the control group who did not change their diet but were instead given social support. Remarkably, about one-third of the patients in the dietary support group had met the criteria for remission of major depression, compared to only 8 per cent in the control group. This was a hugely significant reduction.

Although only sixty-seven patients took part in it, there's no question that this was a highly significant trial, and it's one I expect to see fully replicated in larger sample sizes over the coming years. Researchers are already trying to figure out what exactly it is about the diet that caused such an improvement, but I don't think they'll end up finding just one thing.

Multiple aspects of this diet are beneficial for our mental health. The lack of highly processed food and the presence of wholefoods such as colourful fruit and vegetables will have had a calming effect on the immune system. This would have reduced inflammation, the root cause of many cases of depression. These foods will also have reduced 'leaky gut' and the amount of toxic LPSs that are getting into the bloodstream. Oily fish is rich in omega-3 fats, and we know they can have a positive effect on our mood. In addition, the Mediterranean diet contains a highly diverse set of foods that will have an extremely positive effect on the gut microbiome, which in turn will send beneficial messages up to the brain.

DIVERSITY RULES

Although we're still trying to understand exactly what a healthy microbiome looks like, one thing that's become clear is that diversity in your diet and so in your gut bacteria is crucial. The more diverse your gut bacteria, the healthier you'll be and the more psychologically resilient. By bolstering our gut bugs and increasing their diversity, we can help protect ourselves from the impact of Micro Stress Doses (MSDs).

Unfortunately, all the evidence suggests that modern life is especially bad at supplying us with diversity (see box on p.141). Recently, some staggering statistics have been coming out of Tanzania, where detailed studies have been carried out on populations that are still relatively untouched by modernity. The Hadza community is one such tribe. Analyses of their microbiomes suggest that we in the West have lost up to 50 per cent of our gut-bug diversity. People in the Hadza community even have strains of bugs that are entirely absent in most of our gut microbiomes. As Martin Blaser theorized in his brilliant *Missing Microbes*, those missing gut bugs may be a big part of the reason why so many chronic non-communicable diseases like type 2 diabetes, obesity and inflammatory bowel disease, as well as food allergies and intolerances, are on the rise.

How has this happened? It turns out that these tribespeople, who still live the hunter-gatherer lifestyle we all once did, eat an incredible diversity of plant food. They have access to over 8,000 different plants and, on average, eat around 2,000 of these over the course of their lifetimes. Most of the average Western diet, meanwhile, comes from just three plants: corn, rice and wheat. The Hadza's diverse diet provides them with bucketloads of fibre, which is exactly what our gut bugs want and need. Amazingly, they consume about ten times the amount of fibre we do. This amounts to between 100g and 150g a day – up to forty times the amount you'll get from a bowl of so-called 'high-fibre' bran flakes.

EATING THE ALPHABET

Eating a diverse diet rich in fibre is one of the single best things we can do to live a more stress-free life. A diverse diet means a diverse and resilient microbiome. If we increase the variety of vegetables, low-glycaemic fruits (such as blueberries and cherries) and fibre-rich foods such as beans and legumes in our diet, we're increasing the amount of fibre we're eating. This will encourage the growth of different and happy gut bugs, sending signals to your brain that everything is good.

Eating the alphabet over thirty days will encourage such diversity. It will mean you'll be getting lots of different kinds of crucial fibres, including inulin, which is found in leeks, onions, garlic and artichokes, and pectin, which is found in apples. A diverse diet will also be rich in a class of special nutrients called polyphenols. These help increase the growth of beneficial bacteria; one of the most polyphenolic-rich foods – berries – are a daily staple for the Hadza. Cocoa is known for being rich in a particular group of polyphenols called flavonoids which encourage the growth of healthy bacteria.

Put up a chart in your kitchen and see if you can eat the alphabet every month. I think a realistic goal is to aim for twenty-six different plant foods a month.

Please use the chart overleaf as a guide only – feel free to tweak! The goal is to have at least twenty-six different plant foods every single month. Why not involve your friends and family in this as well?

If you are not used to eating this amount of fibre each day, I would suggest that you build up slowly to allow your gut – and your gut bugs – to adapt!

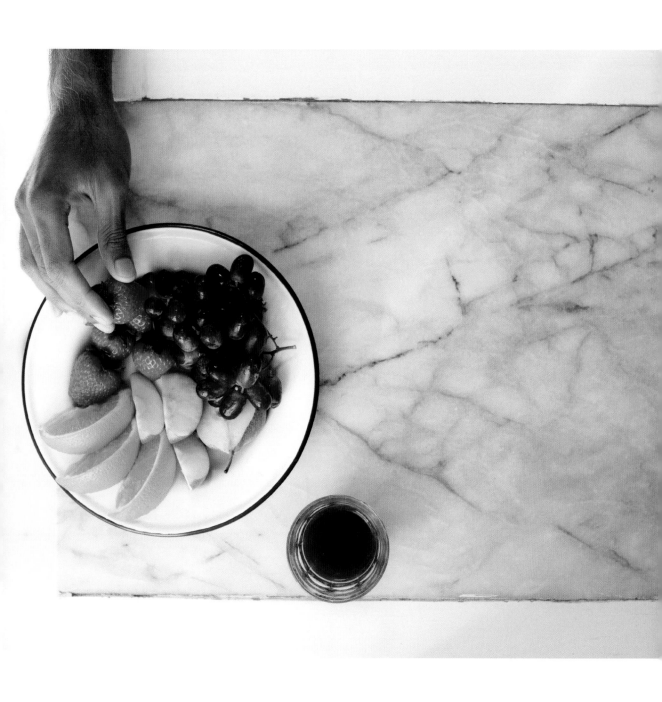

A　ASPARAGUS, APPLES, ARTICHOKES　✓　NOTES

B　BANANAS, BERRIES, BOK CHOY, BROCCOLI, BRUSSELS SPROUTS, BEETROOT, BLACK BEANS, BRAZIL NUTS　✓　NOTES

C　COCOA, CHICKPEAS, CABBAGE, CELERY, CELERIAC, CAULIFLOWER, CHARD, CARROTS, CUCUMBERS, CASHEW NUTS　✓　NOTES

D　DANDELION GREENS, DILL　✓　NOTES

E　EGGPLANT (AUBERGINE), EDAMAME BEANS　✓　NOTES

F　FENNEL, FAVA (OR BROAD) BEANS　✓　NOTES

G　GINGER, GARLIC, GARDEN PEAS　✓　NOTES

H　HERBS, HABANERO PEPPERS, HARICOT BEANS, HAZELNUTS　✓　NOTES

I　ICEBERG LETTUCE　✓　NOTES

J　JALAPEÑO PEPPERS, JERUSALEM ARTICHOKES　✓　NOTES

K　KALE, KIDNEY BEANS, KIWI FRUIT　✓　NOTES

L　LENTILS, LETTUCE, LEMONGRASS, LEEKS　✓　NOTES

M　MARROW, MUSHROOMS　✓　NOTES

N   NETTLES, NECTARINES, NUTS

NOTES

O   OKRA, OLIVES, ONIONS

NOTES

P   PARSNIPS, PARSLEY, PEPPERS, PEAS, PAPRIKA, PUMPKIN, POTATOES, PINTO BEANS

NOTES

Q   QUINCE, QUINOA

NOTES

R   RADICCHIO, RHUBARB, RED ONIONS, ROCKET, ROSEMARY, RADISHES, RASPBERRIES

NOTES

S   SEAWEED, SWEET POTATOES, SQUASH, SPINACH, SHALLOTS, STRAWBERRIES

NOTES

T   TURNIPS, TOMATOES

NOTES

U   URAD DAAL

NOTES

V   VANILLA

NOTES

W   WASABI, WATERCRESS, WATER CHESTNUTS, WATERMELON

NOTES

X   XIGUA (CHINESE WATERMELON). THESE ARE VERY RARE, PARTICULARLY IN THE UK.

NOTES

Y   YAMS, YELLOW LENTILS

NOTES

Z   ZUCCHINI (COURGETTE)

NOTES

IRRITABLE BOWEL SYNDROME

Irritable bowel syndrome (IBS) affects up to 20 per cent of the UK population and can be a major cause of distress and disability for the people who suffer it. The symptoms can be widespread and include abdominal pain and cramps, bloating and nausea. Many sufferers experience a sudden, overwhelming urge to go to the toilet and, when they do, it's often diarrhoea. Others get horrendously constipated.

I recently treated a patient whose IBS was so severe it ended up derailing her career. Belinda was a researcher at a broadcast company and the layout of her office was such that she had to pass her boss's desk every time she wanted to use the bathroom. She became so distressed by the number of times she had to walk past him she quit. I decided to put her on what is called a 'low FODMAP' diet under the supervision of a nutrition professional. FODMAP stands for 'fermentable oligosaccharides, disaccharides, monosaccharides and polyols' – they're easily fermentable sugars that are found in certain foods, like leeks, garlic, onions as well as apples, bread and milk. Over the past few years it has become clear that eating large amounts of FODMAPs can cause symptoms to flare up in some IBS sufferers. By removing them from Belinda's diet, I saw a quick improvement.

But there's a problem with restricting FODMAPs for too long. It means we're not giving our gut bugs the healthy foods they need. While it controlled Belinda's symptoms, every time we tried to introduce healthy but high FODMAP foods back into Belinda's diet her symptoms would get worse. It was only when I added meditation and deep breathing to her routine that she was able to start eating the alphabet again. Belinda is still doing well to this day, but it was only when I tackled her diet and her stress that her threshold moved. That calmed the whole system down, she dropped beneath her stress threshold, and then I was able to start expanding her diet, which gave her more resilience and a greater buffer against MSDs.

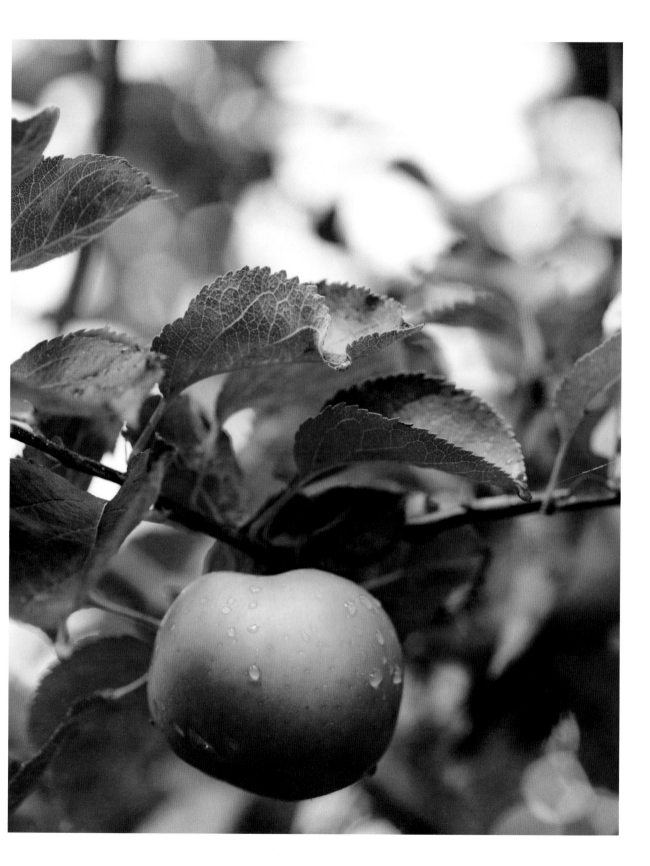

SEVEN FOOD-RELATED TIPS THAT WILL IMPROVE YOUR GUT HEALTH

1. **When you are eating out, try something new from the menu.** This will help to diversify your diet and help you *eat the alphabet*.

2. **Look for new foods to buy.** When in the supermarket, be on the lookout for a type of fibre-rich plant food that you have never tried before.

3. **Give yourself a twelve-hour window every day without food,** for example, if you finish your evening meal at 7 p.m., don't have your breakfast until 7 a.m. the next day. (See p. 187 for more information on time-restricted eating.)

4. **Try to limit eating snacks between meals – research suggests that our gut bugs thrive when they get a break from food.** A new set of gut bugs comes in and cleans up the gut wall.

5. **Skip a meal now and again.** We do not *need* to eat three meals a day. Many of us do very well on only two. If you're not feeling hungry, don't eat. It is not harmful to miss breakfast, or dinner, now and again. If you are on medications that can lower your blood sugar (e.g. gliclazide for type 2 diabetes) it is best to discuss with your doctor.

6. **Eat fermented foods such as kimchi, sauerkraut or kefir.** These are foods that introduce beneficial bacteria into your body, thus improving your gut health.

7. **Avoid artificial sweeteners** – research suggests that they are detrimental to your gut bugs.

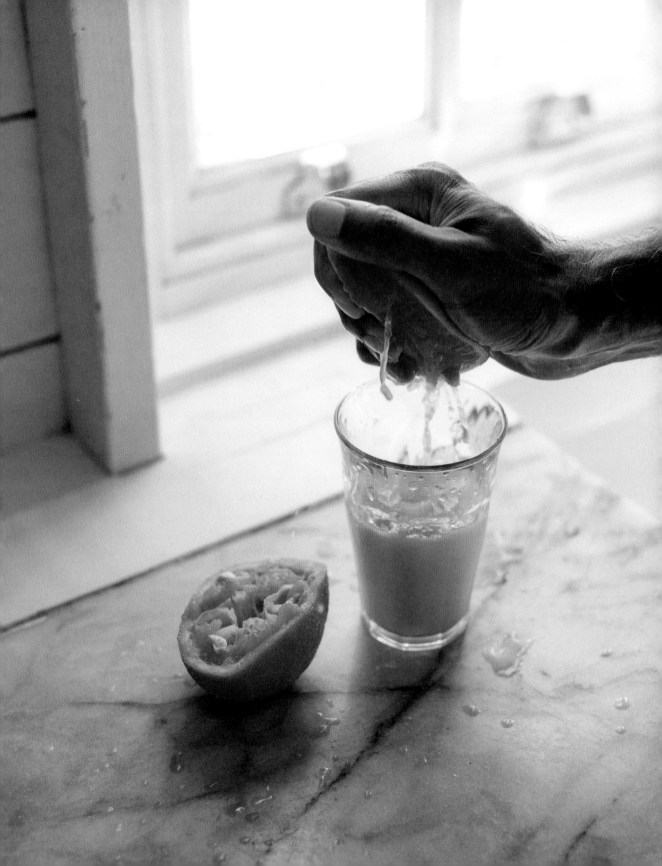

PROBIOTICS

Although eating a more diverse diet is the best thing we can do to ensure a thriving microbiome, it's also possible to introduce 'good' bacteria directly into the gut by taking probiotic supplements. These bacteria, although not taking up permanent residence in our guts, help encourage the growth of beneficial bugs as they are passing through. While research on probiotics is exploding, it's important to stress that much more work is needed to confirm exactly which strains are helpful for which complaints. In addition, there is a huge variation in quality between manufacturers.

Recent research powerfully suggests that such interventions can affect the way our brains function. One 2017 study showed that pregnant women who were given a particularly well-studied organism, *Lactobacillus rhamnosus*, as a probiotic had significantly lower rates of depression and anxiety after they'd given birth. Another test involved twenty-two men being given a probiotic capsule of a bacterium called *Bifidobacterium longum*. After being exposed to a stressor, they ended up with lower levels of the stress response hormone cortisol, felt less anxious and had an enhanced capacity to memorize material, as compared with a control group. This was a small study but hopefully it will soon be repeated on a larger group. Another exciting experiment is looking at whether the administration of probiotics can help treat US veterans who are suffering from post-traumatic stress disorder (PTSD).

SEVEN NON-FOOD TIPS TO IMPROVE
YOUR GUT HEALTH

1. **Only take antibiotics when absolutely necessary.** If you do need to take them, I would always recommend taking a probiotic such as *Saccharomyces boulardii* at the same time. Note, French hospitals have been giving probiotics with antibiotics for years. It amazes me that we haven't yet followed suit in the UK.

2. **Avoid non-essential medications.** We are learning that many drugs, including paracetamol and the proton pump inhibitors which reduce our stomach's acid production, can have a negative impact on the microbiome.

3. **Lower your stress.** Too much stress has a negative impact on your gut bugs and can increase the leakiness of your gut. The tips in this book are designed to help you with this.

4. **Get adequate sleep.** Good-quality, refreshing sleep is good for your microbiome.

5. **Don't try to be 'too' clean.** A modern obsession with hygiene means that we are nuking many of our gut bugs with constant use of antibacterial sprays and hand-washing.

6. **Don't over-exercise.** Too much exercise (see p. 160) can be detrimental to your gut health.

7. **Speak to a healthcare professional about whether you would benefit from taking a high-quality probiotic supplement.**

Chapter 8
MAKE EXERCISE WORK FOR YOU

What I'm about to say might seem a little surprising after we've spent so long discovering how damaging stress can be, but a little bit of stress can actually be a good thing. It's via our stress response that exercise transfers its benefits to the body. We stress our muscles at the gym and they grow back stronger. Exercise is one of the best ways to pull yourself out of a damaging stress state that's been caused by too many Micro Stress Doses (MSDs). Over time, it will help you bring down the levels of stress hormones such as cortisol and adrenaline and reduce inflammation. Exercise, when done in the right dose, sends your brain information that you are thriving.

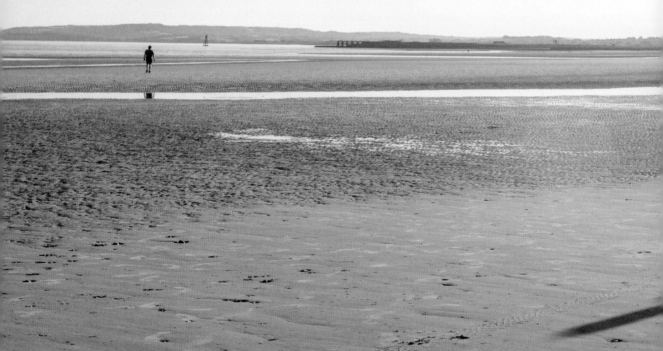

But it is possible to over-exercise. Too much sweat and panting can drive up inflammation, put your immune system on high alert and cause your body more stress. Exercise is information. Too long on the treadmill and it's as if your body starts thinking, 'What's going on out there? She can't stop running! There must be some sort of war on!' It switches you into stress state. I understand that this isn't the most useful health advice you've ever received. So how do we find the balance? Well, in order to grasp the complex relationship between exercise and stress, we must first take a peek at the laws of dose response.

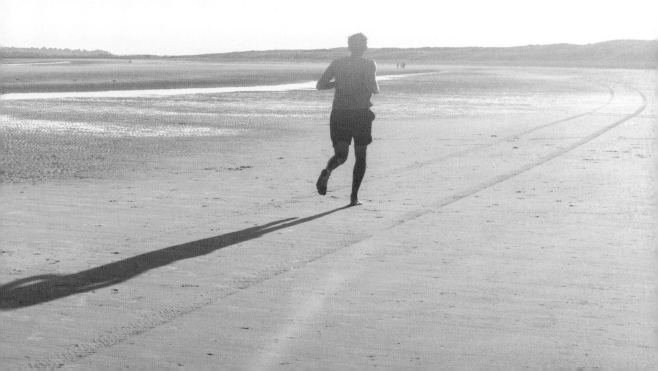

HORMESIS

There's an important concept in medical science called hormesis. It was first discussed in the context of stress nearly twenty years ago by Dr Edward Calabrese, a professor in public health at the University of Massachusetts. It relates to the fact that exposure to a small amount of a stressor can actually do the body good, while exposure to a large amount can be detrimental. For instance, a small amount of cortisol helps your brain work better, improving the function of your hippocampus, the memory centre in your brain. You might have an exam or a meeting with your boss and you're a bit nervous but find this stress helps you pull things from your brain that you haven't thought about in a long time. This is a perfect example of stress behaving as it should, nudging you into a higher level of performance during the fleeting moments when you feel you might be in danger. But when that same process is prolonged, the cortisol that made your hippocampus work so much better instead damages it, which can lead to a multitude of problems, not least the development of memory problems as we get older, including Alzheimer's.

You can also view exercise through the lens of hormesis. With the right intensity and in the right dose, working out can be a phenomenal antidote to stress. If we've had a bad day, a burst of activity in the gym or on the squash court or a jog can leave us feeling relieved and refreshed. But it can also harm us. One of my best friends has two young kids and works in a very busy job in IT. His way of managing the stresses of a work week and a young family include going for a jog. He knows when he jogs for half an hour, twice a week, he can cope with all the other problems in his life. When he gets his jogs in, he performs well at work, he gets on with his wife and he's a great dad. But three weeks ago an old schoolfriend was in town and invited him to go on a two-and-a-half-hour run. So the next Sunday, that's just what he did. And it killed him. For the next two or

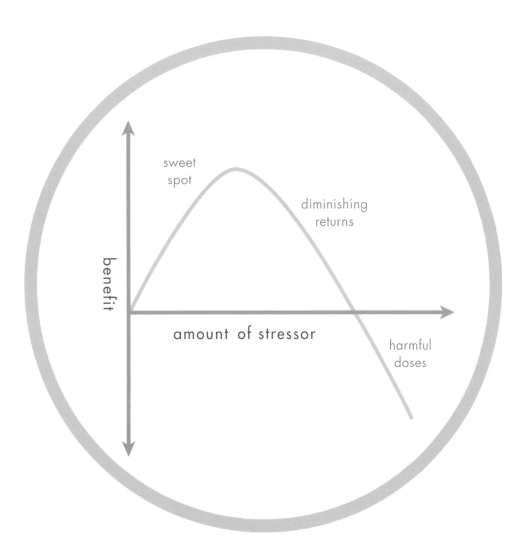

three days he snapped at his kids and reacted more negatively to what his wife was telling him. He realized, on reflection, that it was too much for him. Half an hour was a bullet of calm but, by doing five times the amount of that same form of exercise, it became a cannonball of stress. It stressed his biology, which stressed his mood, which stressed his social environment, and all that turned back on him and caused yet more stress.

HOW EXERCISE FIGHTS STRESS

Study after study has shown that the right amount of exercise can be incredibly beneficial for a variety of psychological conditions, including depression and anxiety. One even found that regular workouts can be more effective for treating depression than medication. Exercise ameliorates stress in multiple ways. One of the major problems with the human stress response is that it evolved to put us in fight-or-flight mode, which prepares us for dealing with the kinds of serious physical problems we'd have encountered tens of thousands of years ago. But today's stressors are very rarely physical (as much as we might want them to be) – we won't do much good by physically assaulting or running away from our email inbox. But that's what our bodies are primed to do. Exercise gives it what it needs and is expecting: a physical workout that helps ease us out of fight-or-flight mode.

It also helps the body practise moving more fluidly in and out of the stress state. When we exercise, levels of various 'stress' hormones such as cortisol and adrenaline go up in the short term. The same hormones rise when we're stressed through other means. Regular physical activity teaches our stress response system how to recover more efficiently and means our stress responses can operate much more efficiently when we're being attacked by our daily MSDs. Exercise also seems to help us reorganize our brains so that they're more resistant to MSDs. In 2013 researchers at Princeton University found that mice which exercised showed large increases in a brain chemical called GABA, which is known to help switch the brain into its calm state. Remarkably, they even showed an increase in the brain cell activity that helps dampen down anxiety and lessen the effects of an overactive stress response.

Next time you're feeling overwhelmed or anxious, try doing a quick burst of exercise. It can be a quick two minutes of bodyweight exercises (such as press-ups or lunges), dancing to your favourite tunes for a few minutes, ten minutes of a high-intensity workout or a brisk walk around the block. Once you have done it, observe how stressed you are feeling, compared to before. Almost always, your stress levels will have gone down.

TELOMERES

There is another important mechanism by which exercise can help reduce the impact of stress on the body, and that's through its effect on our telomeres. Deep inside our cells are chromosomes which carry all our genetic material. If you imagine chromosomes as being like very tiny shoelaces, telomeres are the protective caps you find at the end of them. If your telomeres are damaged, your chromosomes can start to fray, which is a key sign of cellular ageing. Cellular ageing means our bodies are ageing!

Research by scientists such as Nobel Prize-winners Dr Elizabeth Blackburn and Dr Elissa Epel suggests that various lifestyle factors may keep us young by preventing the shortening of our telomeres. They argue that low stress levels, good-quality sleep, a diet full of minimally processed wholefoods and time spent in nature all help.

But exercise seems to play a role as well. A 2010 study demonstrated that stressed-out women who carried out vigorous exercise had longer, more healthy telomeres than their inactive, stressed-out counterparts. Incredibly, this effect could be seen with only fourteen minutes of vigorous daily activity. The researchers concluded that 'vigorous physical activity appears to protect those experiencing high stress by buffering its relationship with telomeres'. The key take-home from this and other studies is that we ought to reduce the amount of time we sit, as well as aim for moderate amounts of physical activity every week.

HOW TO FIND YOUR PERFECT DOSE

Your perfect dose of exercise will depend on the state of the rest of your life. You should always be asking yourself whether your body needs a restorative workout or an intense one. If you've been super busy at work and didn't sleep particularly well, it may be that you're closer to your stress threshold and would benefit from a restorative form of exercise such as yoga or Pilates rather than pounding away on the treadmill. It's crucial to start listening to your body. When you do, you'll start to become more in tune with what kind of workout your body needs.

Signs that you might be over-exercising include:

- Inability to sleep at night following a vigorous workout

- Sleeping too much, compared to your norm, and still feeling exhausted

- Waking up with your heart racing the day after an intense workout

- Feeling exhausted for the rest of the day following a workout

- Feeling irritable and moody after an increase in the intensity of your exercise

- Frequently getting ill (for example, coughs and colds)

- Impaired heart-rate variability (see p. 169)

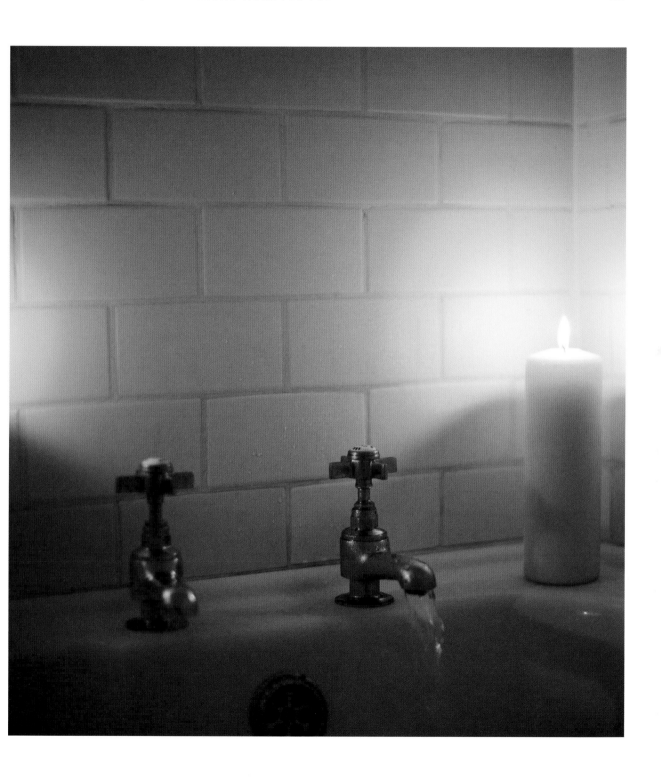

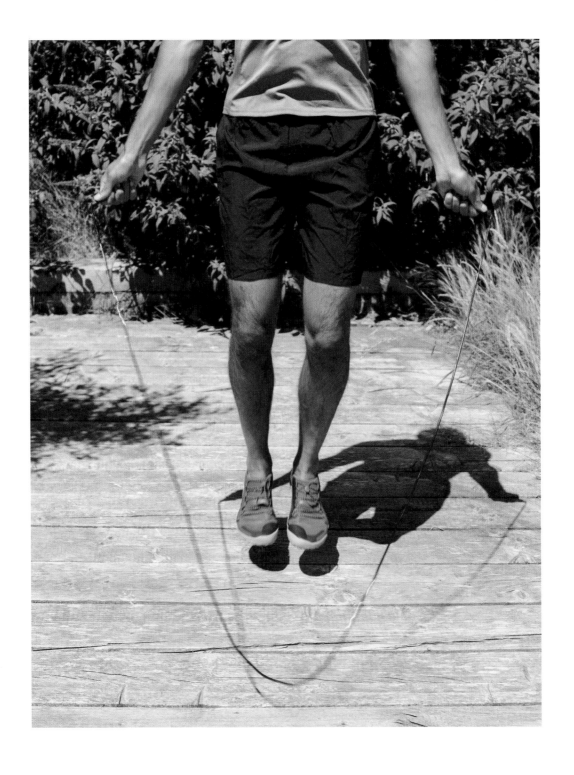

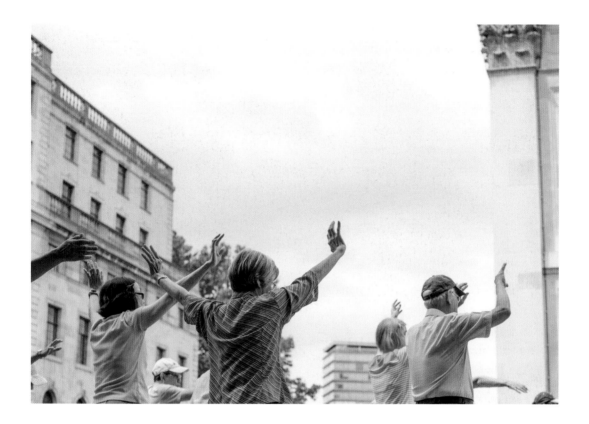

YOUR DAILY EXERCISE PRESCRIPTION

I'd like you to do a form of stress-busting exercise every single day. Physical activity is the perfect antidote to stress. Stress doesn't take a day off, so neither should physical activity. It can be as simple as a ten-minute walk at lunchtime, a high-intensity interval session or a long one-hour jog – you choose! The key is to move your body as much as possible each day, in any way you like. Importantly, pay attention to how you feel afterwards to ensure that you start to tune into your body and how you are feeling. Try and make sure that you are doing the right kind of activity that is in harmony with the rest of your lifestyle.

BURN THE STRESS AWAY

Over the past few years there's been some incredible research carried out on 'hyperthermia', or the increase of core body temperature. It's been found that if you raise your core temperature to 38.5° C – which is the sort of level you'd reach when hot and sweaty with fever – for about an hour or so, it can reduce stress and raise mental function. Studies of sauna therapy have shown such treatment can alleviate the symptoms of depression, while research in Japan found that a sauna a day, for five days a week, over a course of four weeks reduced the stress state and increased the thrive state.

A study of Bikram Yoga (a form of 'hot yoga') found that it significantly reduced the symptoms of depression. Heat, which can be a form of 'good stress' on the body, and exercise, such as yoga, both induce the release of beta-endorphins, which help relieve pain and elevate mood. Could it be that the beneficial stress induced by heat and the beneficial stress induced by yoga have their effects magnified when you put them together?

My experience with a fifty-five-year-old patient called Simon has led me to strongly suspect something like this is going on. He'd been struggling with his mood, had not got on well with therapy and had been on multiple antidepressants, but found that none of them worked for him. He was the sort of patient who would come in every few months frustrated that his mood was flat and that we just weren't getting anywhere. Then one day he met a woman on a dating website who invited him to a hot-yoga class. Remarkably, for several days after the session, he felt elated and happy. I assumed that this was simply because he'd found love. But they soon stopped seeing each other, Simon joined a different hot-yoga class and reports experiencing a significant and sustained improvement in mood.

Why not try hot yoga for yourself and see how it makes you feel? If hot yoga doesn't appeal, what about spending some time in a sauna or steam room? You can even try doing some light stretches or yoga moves while in there, if you have room and it's not too busy!

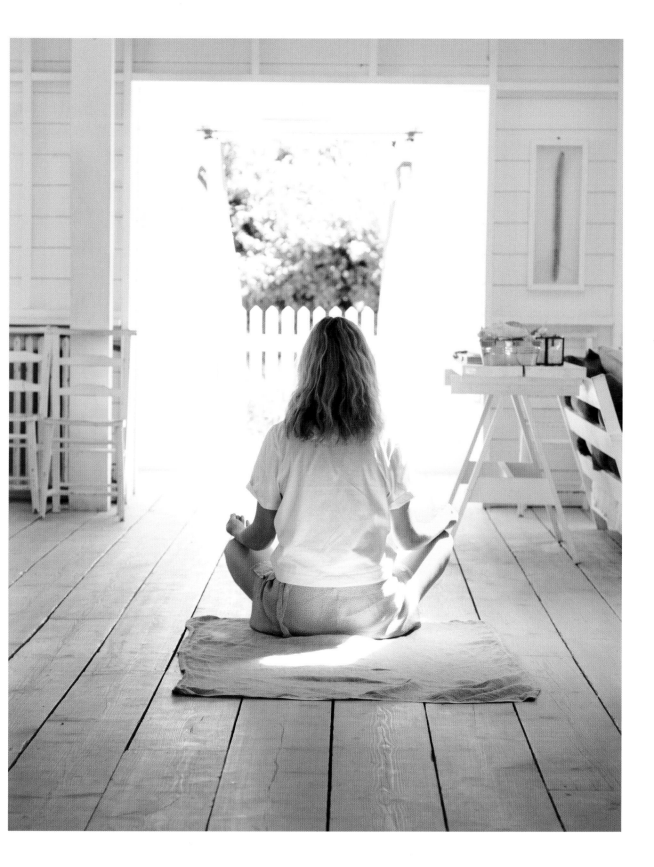

SEVEN GREAT WORKOUTS YOU
MAY NOT HAVE CONSIDERED

1. **Indoor climbing:** Exercise that demands concentration, which forces us to switch off.

2. **Open-water swimming:** There's something incredibly therapeutic about being in open water, such as oceans, lakes and rivers. Even if you are unable to swim regularly in an open-water setting, indoor swimming still has tremendous benefits. One of the best things about swimming, whether open water or indoor, is that you can't have your phone with you, so it forces you to switch off from the stresses of the outside world.

3. **T'ai chi or yoga in the forest or local park.**

4. **Skipping:** A free and quick way to burn off excess 'stress energy' – all you need is a skipping rope.

5. **A run in nature:** If you already run regularly in urban areas, try switching it up sometimes with a run in nature.

6. **Nordic walking – a four-wheel-drive version of walking:** It is a whole-body workout using your feet as well as your arms, by using poles.

7. **Ground living:** Try to spend more time on the floor, kneeling, squatting or balancing on yoga balls when you eat, read or watch TV to counter all that time we spend slumped over computers.

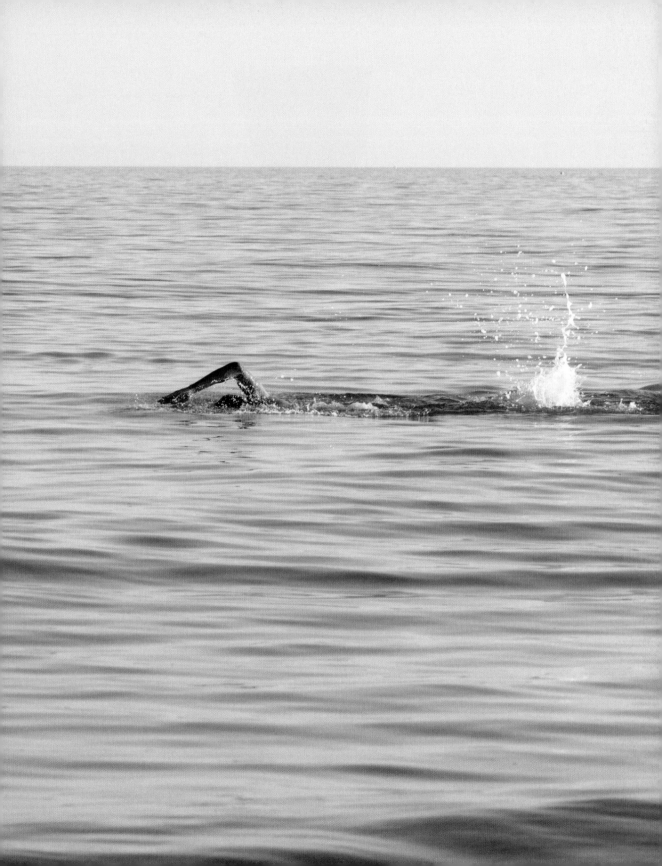

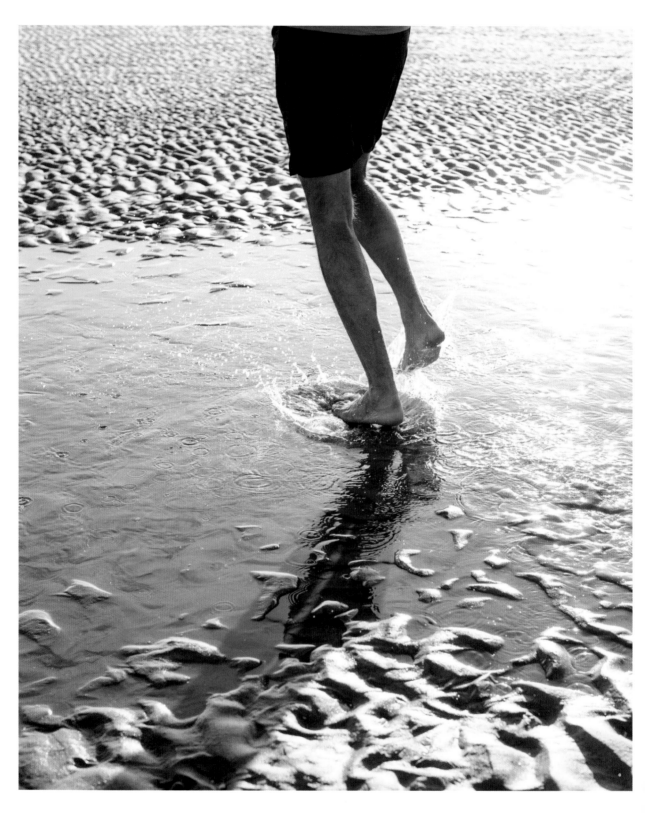

HEART-RATE VARIABILITY

People often think that the heart should beat like a metronome, following a strict, clock-like rhythm. Surprisingly, this is incorrect. The amount of time taken from one heartbeat to the next should vary. When we're functioning well and are comfortably distant from our stress threshold, we have high heart-rate variability (HRV). From one beat to the next there's a change in rhythm and strength. It's a reflection that the body is capable of adapting to a constantly changing environment. I often think about it as a marker of resilience – our body's ability to cope with stress.

But when we're overdoing things, this variability goes. Low HRV has been linked to multiple poor health outcomes, such as all-cause mortality and heart disease. There are many different things that can lower HRV including infections, temperature, inflammation as well as traumatic Macro Stress Doses. However, for the vast majority of us, what affects our HRV the most on a daily basis is the relentless bombardment of MSDs that leave us feeling drained. Low HRV indicates that our body is in stress state and not thrive.

1 second   1 second   1 second   1 second

Low HRV (stress state).
Time between each heartbeat is constant.

0.85 seconds   0.92 seconds   1.34 seconds   1.12 seconds

High HRV (thrive state).
Time between each heartbeat is constantly changing.

It's becoming increasingly common to see professional athletes, as well as weekend warriors, using HRV apps such as HRV4Training or Elite HRV to help them determine what sort of training they should be doing. A high HRV indicates that they're relaxed and have low levels of stress and can benefit from going hard. A low HRV suggests that the body has taken the hit from multiple MSDs and is in need of rest, recovery and relaxation, so they might try yoga or stretching, or even give the workout a miss.

I found using an HRV app absolutely fascinating. So many factors negatively impacted my readings, among them eating out, caffeine, a poor night's sleep, alcohol and travel. A friend of mine, Alessandro Ferretti, studies HRV and religiously tracks his rate with medical-grade equipment. When he watched *Masterchef Australia*, with its genial and encouraging hosts, he found it relaxing and enjoyable and his HRV reflected this. But when he watched *Masterchef USA*, with Gordon Ramsay effing and blinding, he found it so irritating his HRV went down!

These apps have also helped in the surgery. I recently saw a forty-eight-year-old patient, Andrew, who was a tech enthusiast and came armed with his own HRV readings. I decided to have a detailed look at his data. What I found was eye-opening. Every Wednesday afternoon Andrew had to run a team meeting at his firm of corporate headhunters. Because of the stress he'd endured that day, he'd often drink half a bottle of wine on Wednesday evenings. This would inevitably cause him to have disrupted sleep, which would lead him to wake up groggy and tired on Thursday. To compensate for his ill mood, he'd gorge on sweet treats and caffeine throughout the day and become progressively more tired and moody. He'd literally be counting the minutes until the end of the working week; Thursday and Friday were almost unbearable. He'd get through at least a bottle of wine on Friday nights and spend the rest of the weekend recovering.

Andrew's data showed that, after he consumed alcohol on Wednesday evening, his HRV readings plummeted, which meant that on Thursday mornings he'd be right up against his stress threshold. This helped explain why those days were so tricky for him. Armed with this information, we planned a strategy. On Wednesdays, he would no longer go back home, slump on the sofa and crack open a bottle of red wine. Instead, he found a local yoga class and would pop in on the way home from work. By making this single change to his routine, his working week was transformed. He would wake up on Thursday mornings feeling refreshed. He'd eat fewer sugary snacks and felt less of a need to drink caffeine. He also felt calmer and more productive at work. Over the next few weeks he fed back to me that Thursdays and Fridays were now his most enjoyable work days. He also told me that on Friday nights he would no longer drink a whole bottle of wine. He would either drink a single glass, or occasionally abstain, as he felt less stressed at the end of his week.

By empowering himself with this knowledge and seeing the impact on his biology, Andrew was motivated to change his behaviour. When I saw him two months later he was beaming. His workload had not changed – he was still being hit by multiple MSDs throughout the day – but what had changed was his capacity to absorb those MSDs. Over the course of just a few weeks his energy levels had increased, he felt less stressed and his mood had improved.

I'm sure you'll have had mornings when you've woken up feeling great and rested. You march on into the day and deal with all those MSDs like a swordsman of old, batting them away as they come flying at you. You'll very likely have a high HRV reading on days like this. Contrast that feeling to the times you've woken up a bit late, felt groggy, needed a gallon of caffeine and everything seemed to involve a lot of effort and stress. I'd bet, on a day like that, your HRV reading would be low. You would be very close to your personal stress threshold and it wouldn't take much to push you over it. I'm not advocating that you meticulously track your readings every hour. I use a simple app once a day in the morning to give me an idea of what my status is for the day and to guide me in my exercise choices.

ELEVEN WAYS TO INCREASE HRV

These are just suggestions. You don't need to do them all. Pick a few that you think you can implement in your life.

1. **Get enough sleep – 'enough' sleep should leave you feeling refreshed and rested.** Seven to nine hours seems to be the sweet spot for most.

2. **Eat your last meal of the day at least three hours before going to bed** (see p. 189 for more details).

3. **Prioritize exercise.** Do a form of strength training at least twice a week and move as much as possible each day.

4. **Practise deep breathing,** the 3–4–5 breath and alternate-nostril breathing for five to ten minutes every morning (see pp. 246–7).

5. **Eat a diet rich in whole, unprocessed foods** (see Eating the Alphabet on p. 144).

6. **Do some form of regular yoga practice.** I like patients to do ten minutes a day. Weekly classes can be helpful as well, but I find doing less but more often is a much better way of reducing stress and raising HRV levels.

7. Practise meditation.

8. Listen to relaxing music.

9. Go for a walk in nature.

10. Take up t'ai chi.

11. **Do a daily practice of gratitude** (see p. 46).

RELEASING STRESS FROM THE BODY

Because our bodies store stress, we can also use our bodies to release it. In this, we're no different from animals such as polar bears, who are seen vigorously shaking or trembling after traumatic incidents in order to discharge feelings of stress.

- DO ONE MINUTE OF INTENSE ACTIVITY. This will help your body 'process' the stress that has built up in your system. It could be twenty press-ups, some star jumps or even a brisk walk.

- DO SOME FORM OF BODY WORK SUCH AS DEEP-TISSUE MASSAGE OR MYOFASCIAL RELEASE. Fascia is the cling-film-type substance that surrounds our tissues and organs which helps reduce friction and pain as we move. Myofascial release aims to stretch this cling film out. It's thought many of us 'store' our stresses in our bodies, which is why many people have dramatic emotional responses to deep-tissue work or therapies such as myofascial release. A regular form of body work may help you discharge your stress.

- DO TWO MINUTES OF DEEP BREATHING. This helps to change your physiology immediately and give your brain the signals to put you into a thrive state. (For more on breathing, see p. 245.)

- HAVE A GOOD CRY. Everyone tends to feel better after crying and, if you are highly stressed, it can often be easier to take full deep breaths after a good cry.

- LAUGH UNCONTROLLABLY FOR A FEW MINUTES. Watch your favourite comedian on YouTube or have a giggle with your friends. This helps to release endorphins that can reduce stress.

- PRACTISE YOGA. Stretching out the muscles, focusing on the breath and quietening the mind can be hugely beneficial.

- TRY PRIMAL SCREAMING. Although we don't have robust scientific evidence on this, I have seen many patients who report that this technique can be a great stress reliever. The idea is to scream at a comfortably loud volume in order to release your anger and stress. Ideally, you would do this with the lower register of your voice and the sound should come from your belly and not the throat. It is best to do this in a safe environment like your house and some like to do it into a pillow to muffle some of the volume. Some patients report additional benefits from doing it in a guided group session. It may sound rather unusual but if you struggle with stress it is certainly worth a try.

- TRY REFLEXOLOGY. Studies have shown that this gentle and relaxing therapy can help reduce levels of the stress hormone cortisol. Many patients have reported back to me that reflexology helps lower their stress levels and improve their sleep quality.

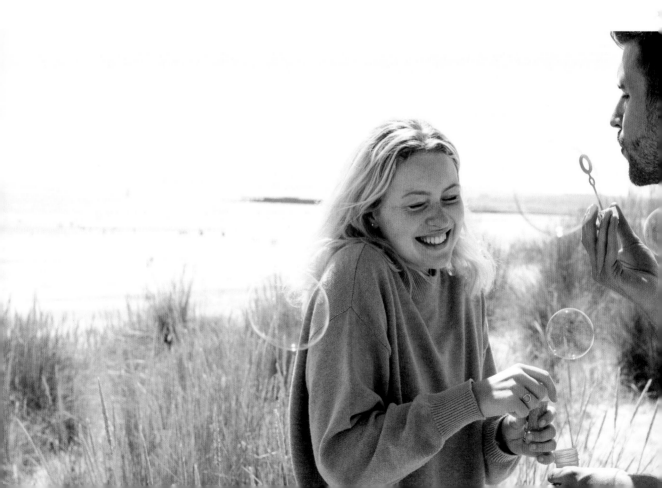

Chapter 9
RESET YOUR RHYTHM

Our biological systems are a bit like an orchestra that's being led by an astonishingly precise conductor. Whereas a musical orchestra has its strings, brass, percussion and horns, we have digestion, muscular strength, liver function and our sleep cycles. The internal rhythms that our bodies live by have been finely tuned over millions of years. But in the last couple of hundred years, since the advent of artificial light, our bodily rhythms have been knocked out of time. It's as if there are now two conductors, one that's trying to get the orchestra to play Mozart, the other to play Eminem. These rhythms we live by are information. Make that information chaotic and the body will respond by switching into stress state.

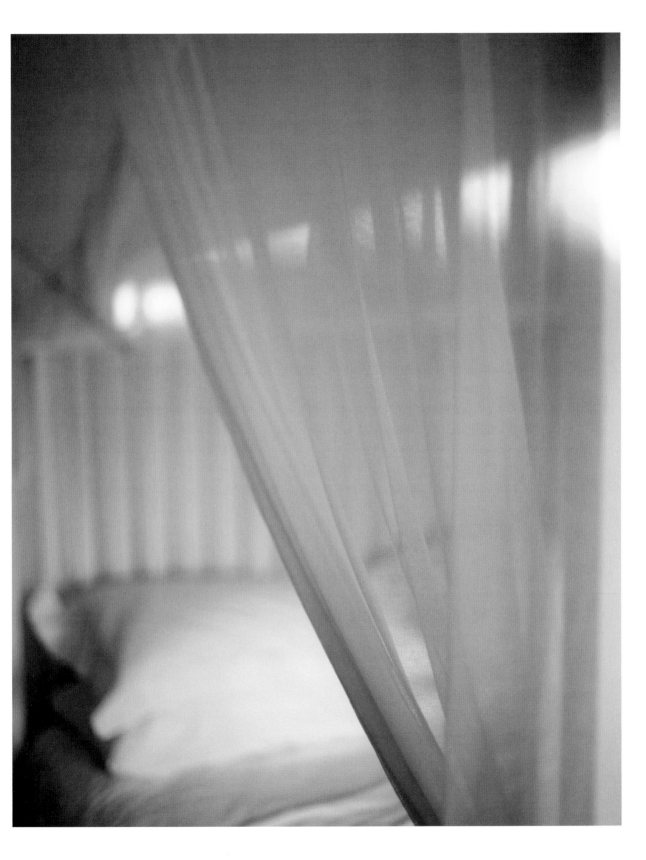

THE MYTH OF THE NIGHT OWL

Perhaps the most well-known internal rhythm is the circadian – the one that wakes us up and sends us to sleep. There's a widespread belief that people possess one of two different kinds of circadian rhythms, with some being 'morning larks', bouncing happily out of bed bright and early, while others are 'night owls'. While there is some truth to this, I've come to believe that this difference has been wildly exaggerated.

One of my oldest friends, Andy, spent most of his life convinced he was a night owl. At university, he'd be up late partying at the weekends and lie in recovering every morning. He told everyone he did his best work late at night, when the world was quiet and most people were sleeping. He believed it was his most creative time and, indeed, he did do some really good work after midnight. But the next day he'd struggle to perform well, especially in the afternoons, and would rely heavily on caffeine to get him through. That post-lunch lull convinced him even more that he was just the kind of person who was naturally primed for the hours of dark.

About two years ago Andy became a father. His nights would often be disrupted by his young family, who'd typically wake him up at around 5.30 a.m. He was growing more and more tired and, out of desperation, phoned me for help. He insisted he couldn't go to bed much earlier than he was already because he was a night owl so he'd end up lying there for hours, staring at the ceiling. I told him that if he kept going to bed at one in the morning and waking with his kids at 5.30 a.m. he was going to burn himself out, and fast. I recommended that he start going to bed before ten o'clock, limit his caffeine to the morning, cut out booze in the evenings and stay off his screens for at least an hour before he went to bed. Before I put the phone down I'd managed to persuade him to give this new routine a go for two weeks, then we'd reassess.

Before the first week was out Andy noticed that those afternoon lulls which he'd assumed were just part of his biological make-up didn't happen any more. He also became way more productive during daylight hours and started doing much of his best work in the mornings. He's now decided that he's a lark!

I told Andy's story to Dr Satchidananda Panda, one of the world's premier scientists investigating circadian rhythms, when I was lucky enough to lecture alongside him recently in Iceland. 'I'm a little confused by the whole night-owl and morning-lark thing,' I told him one night, over dinner.

'It's interesting,' he replied. 'We took some of our volunteers on a camping trip where there was little or no artificial light. We found, after a few days of living with natural light rhythms, that the owls and the larks did show a difference. They would go to sleep at different times, but not by very much.'

'How much?' I asked.

'Between about thirty minutes and an hour.'

I've since come to believe that this idea of natural-born owls and larks is, for many of us, a myth. That's not to say there aren't any genetic differences that influence our circadian rhythms. The Nobel Prize-winning researcher Mike Young has shown that some people carry a particular mutation that predisposes them to stay up somewhat later. However, of those that do, we don't know how many are actually impacted by it.

The bottom line is this. Most of us are adopting behaviours that are throwing our circadian rhythms out. Partly, this is a simple consequence of modern urban living. One study found that we're exposed to 10,000 times more light at night today than we were in the 1700s, which can shift the body clock back by up to three hours. In the twenty-first century we stay up later, we eat later, we exercise later and we keep our brains in an active, alert state for longer. We think we're fixing the problem by having lie-ins at the weekend, but waking up at 6 a.m. every weekday then at 9 a.m. at the weekends is like travelling across three time zones. You're giving yourself jet lag. In some people, lie-ins can even trigger migraines. On top of all this, many of us are now working shifts. Rather than realizing we have a problem, lots of us are simply calling ourselves night owls and thinking we've been born this way. In fact, right now, throughout the West, we're living through a sleep-deprivation epidemic.

SLEEP'S STRESS-BUSTING SIGNATURE

If you're not prioritizing your sleep, it's highly likely that you're not getting enough. When we're as time poor as we are these days, sleep tends to be the first thing to be pushed to the side. This is because we just don't realize how much we need it and how much stress a lack of it can cause.

I had a conversation with Professor Matthew Walker*, sleep scientist and author of the bestselling *Why We Sleep*, in which he told me, 'Sleep loss in the brain has a signature that's similar to stress.' When we expose ourselves to a lack of sleep, it expresses itself in the body as a stressor. If you look in the brain, you see a collapse in memory, attention, cognitive function, decision-making capacity and ability to learn new things. In the body, levels of adrenaline, noradrenaline and cortisol increase, inflammatory markers go up, and we become resistant to insulin, which makes it more likely that we will develop type 2 diabetes. Lack of sleep also causes

---

* You can listen to an in-depth conversation that I have with Professor Walker about sleep on my *Feel Better, Live More* podcast at drchatterjee.com/matthewwalker and drchatterjee.com/whywesleep.

hunger and satiety hormones to reverse (see p. 194), meaning that our appetite goes up and we feel less full, making weight gain more likely. If you are lacking in sleep, you're going to be significantly less likely to eat the alphabet because you'll be craving sugary junk food.

And there's an impact at the cellular level. One fascinating study carried out by researchers at the Surrey Sleep Research Centre compared people who had six hours' sleep a night to those who had eight and a half hours' sleep. After just one week, those who had their sleep restricted to six hours a night developed distortions in 711 genes. About half of these – among them genes associated with chronic inflammation, stress, cardiovascular disease and cancer – went up in activity. The other half – associated with having a balanced immune system and a stable metabolism – went down in activity. Sleep deprivation was changing the way the genes expressed themselves. In addition, sleep loss lowers heart-rate variability (a marker for increased stress; see p. 169), is associated with damaged telomeres, which is a key sign of cellular ageing, increases activity in the HPA axis (our stress broadcast service; see p. 16) and negatively impacts the microbiome (see p. 137).

These are just some of the mechanisms through which lack of sleep can put the body into stress state. But it also gives the brain information that things are wrong. This is partly due to its effects on our emotional brain. Researchers have shown that the amygdala, our emotional brain's alarm system, is significantly more reactive when we are sleep deprived. This is why we have such an increased tendency to overreact to negative stimuli. One study found a 60 per cent increase in reactivity when sleep-deprived individuals were exposed to stressful stimuli.

But just as a lack of sleep can radically lower our stress and wellbeing thresholds, getting enough can be amazingly healing. It's been shown to reduce the impact of the most serious stressful and traumatic experiences. If you experience a Macro Stress Dose and your sleep is disturbed afterwards, you're more likely to develop PTSD and depression. Similarly, if you've had a stressful day, one of the most important things you can do is prioritize your sleep that evening.

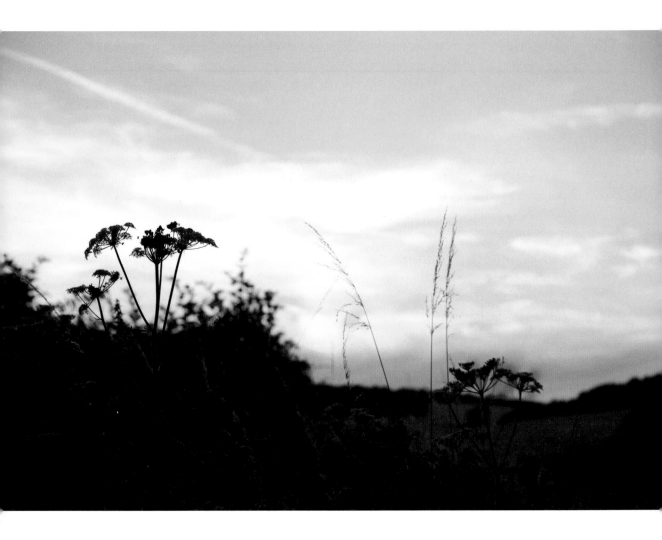

RAISING MELATONIN

In the evening, as it gets dark, a hormone called melatonin is released by the pineal gland, which is located deep inside our brain. We thought for many years that melatonin was simply there to help us fall asleep, but it's now known to have multiple effects on the body. It switches off oxidation – a type of rusting process in the body that can become harmful if it is not kept in check – and helps to dampen down inflammation. But many of us are messing up the timing of our melatonin secretion by exposing ourselves to unnatural light, not least from smartphones and other electronic devices, which are typically held close to the face. Several studies have found that device use before bed can reduce the amount of melatonin you release by more than 50 per cent. If there was a drug that had such a huge and potentially damaging side effect, there'd be warnings printed all over the packet.

At this point, you may well be thinking, 'Well, that's sad for those unlucky people. I can fall asleep just fine after reading on my device.' If you are, I have some disturbing news. Even if you can physically get to sleep after looking at your device, the quality of that sleep is likely to be significantly impaired. You'll lose significant amounts of a critical phase of deep sleep called REM (see p. 192). This will leave you feeling much more tired the following day. Even more worryingly, your melatonin levels may be affected for several days afterwards, even if you stop using your device completely. This is why I always recommend that patients remove temptation by leaving their devices outside the bedroom.

GETTING THE RIGHT LIGHT

A huge part of getting our circadian rhythms moving to the right beat is about getting the right light at the right time. This means exposing ourselves to as much light as possible in the mornings and as little as possible in the evenings. Morning light is blue light and energizes and refreshes. Japanese authorities have recently begun harvesting the power of blue light in extraordinary ways. Japan has one of the highest rates of suicide in the world and many people choose to take their own lives by jumping into the path of oncoming trains. To combat this, blue-light-emitting LEDs have been installed at the end of some station platforms. In some locations where lights have been put in, suicide rates have fallen by a truly remarkable 84 per cent.

In the evening, however, we don't want energizing blue light. Instead, we want to mimic the conditions that our brains evolved in. Candlelight is perfect for re-creating the campfires we would have gathered around and red light is the wavelength that has the least impact on our circadian rhythms. You can buy red light bulbs to use in the home as nightlights or, if you can stretch to it, you could try an electronic solution like Philips Hue, whereby the light automatically changes colour during the day, giving out warm oranges and reds as you dip into the evening. Blue-light-blocking glasses are pretty affordable and wearing them in the evening can be game-changing for many (not least my wife, who puts them on at 8 p.m. and begins to feel drowsy within twenty minutes). My own personal favourites are Blueblox and True Dark. I have even bought some for my kids.

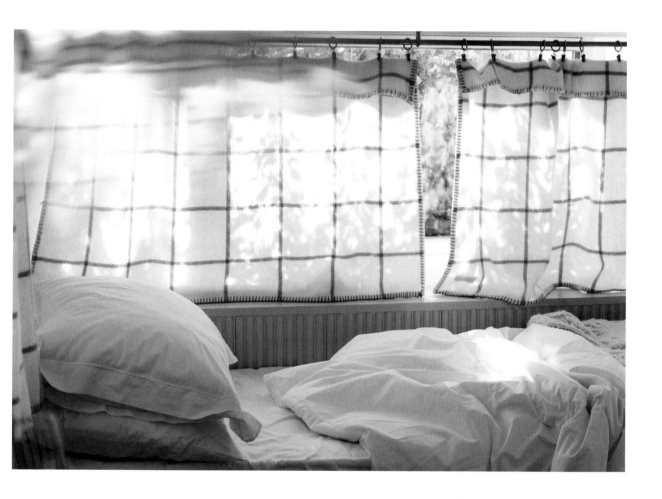

EAT IN RHYTHM

The circadian might be the most famous, but it's by no means the only rhythm our body moves to. Digestion also runs on a daily rhythm. Our bodies are optimized to process food during daylight hours but, again, the reality of modern industrial life means we're living out of sync. In my surgery, I see some of the worst effects of this nutritional de-rhythming in shift workers, a group that has higher than average insulin resistance and more problems with diabetes and cancer. If we want to replicate how our ancestors ate, we should eat the bulk of our food earlier in the day and avoid heavy meals after dark. The old phrase that you should eat breakfast like a king, lunch like a prince and dinner like a pauper has a huge amount of wisdom packed into it.

But I get it – life is complicated: many of us have to work unsocial hours and I realize that changing your eating habits may not be possible. Another solution for getting your eating habits back into rhythm might be to restrict the hours in which you eat. There's recently been some incredible early research on mice done at the Salk Institute in San Diego which has indicated that time-restricted feeding may come with a whole raft of benefits. In the tests, obese mice given a fast-food diet and allowed to eat whenever they wanted seven days a week became morbidly obese. When these obese mice were given the same junk-food diet but were restricted to an eleven-hour eating window, they remained obese – but they became fit. Next, the researcher gave lean mice junk food and let them eat whenever they wanted. Unsurprisingly, they became obese. But intriguingly, when lean mice were given the same fast-food diet but were restricted to eating it in an eleven-hour window they stayed lean and became fit. It was the same diet. It was the same terrible food. The only difference was the mice ate it within a regular, limited window. Finally, the researchers wondered what would happen if they gave lean mice a fast-food diet in a time-restricted manner on weekdays, allowing them to eat as they wished at the weekends, a pattern that is more applicable to the way many of us live today. Even then, the mice stayed lean and fit.

TIME-RESTRICTED EATING

I recommend that *all* of us try to eat our food within a twelve-hour window each day. Of course, you can shorten this eating window if you wish, but for most of us twelve hours is sufficient to reap most of the benefits. Remember, you will, hopefully, be sleeping for about eight of the twelve hours with no food. I regard time-restricted eating to be one of *the* most important things anyone can do for their health.

Outside your eating window, stick to water, herbal tea or black tea or coffee. This strategy can also work well for shift workers (see p. 199).

Research like this is turning our thinking about nutrition on its head. Of course, most of the work so far has been done on mice, and animal results don't necessarily extrapolate to humans. Sadly, the scientists involved have struggled for years to secure funding for human trials, in large part because there is no profit to be made from the outcome. Thankfully, that problem has been partially resolved and early human trials are underway. Early reports are looking very encouraging indeed. In addition, Dr Satchidananda Panda's lab is getting real-world results from people all over the world who are eating this way by tracking their progress on his app, *My Circadian Clock.**

I find these mice studies fascinating, but they simply echo what I've been seeing in my own practice for years. When my patients time-restrict their food intake, I have noticed it help with weight loss, blood-sugar control and general stress levels, as well as digestive disturbances like indigestion and heartburn. I mentioned this concept in my previous book, *The 4 Pillar Plan*, and have been overwhelmed by how many people have contacted me to report similar improvements.

The timing of food intake is also one of the biggest contributors to a healthy HRV reading (see p. 169). Interestingly, many of my friends and patients who religiously monitor their HRV tell me that eating your evening meal early results in a much better reading the following morning. Eating late is a stressor on your body. Even if you don't change what you eat, simply shifting your evening meal back to an earlier time will help move you out of stress state and launch you into thrive state.

---

*You can listen to an in-depth conversation that I have with Dr Panda about this on my *Feel Better, Live More* podcast at drchatterjee.com/panda and drchatterjee.com/trf.

HOW LATE SHOULD YOU EAT YOUR EVENING MEAL?

Evidence is growing that an earlier dinner time is better for multiple different health parameters such as weight, blood-sugar balance and stress levels. I recommend that you try to finish eating at least three hours before going to bed. For example, if ten o'clock is your bedtime, you want to finish your evening meal by seven. You may find this tricky at first if you are not used to it, but stick with it. Within one or two weeks of starting you will find that your body gets used to this change. Patients often report back to me that their heartburn, indigestion and sleep quality improve as well.

If you have to work late, consider taking some food with you or eating dinner in an early evening break.

AVOID LIQUID STRESS

It's long been part of our culture in the West that, when we're stressed, we crack open a beer or have a glass of wine. Because alcohol is a sedative, we've allowed ourselves to believe it helps us sleep. Sure, it knocks you out – you've got your eyes closed and you're unresponsive. But the problem with using alcohol in this way is that it disrupts our sleep, increasing fragmentation, which means we wake up more during the night. Alcohol also blocks out vital and restorative REM sleep. We're having sleep that's not repairing the damage of the stressors of the day. We tend to use alcohol more when we're stressed and, unfortunately, it just ends up causing us more stress.

If you don't sleep as well as you would like, try reducing (or even eliminating) your intake of alcohol for one to two weeks and see what difference it makes. For many, it can be life-changing.

If alcohol is one form of liquid stress, caffeine is another. It might surprise you to learn that, for some of us, a quarter of the cup of coffee you enjoyed at lunchtime is still likely to be in your body come midnight. Everyone knows that it's unwise to have a coffee just before you climb into bed, but that lunchtime coffee is little different from gulping a quarter of an Americano and then turning the light off to get some sleep. Some people can seemingly fall asleep straight after an evening espresso, yet research suggests that, by doing so, they won't enjoy the same quality of restorative sleep. For many, caffeine is a deceptive and hidden source of stress.

Excess caffeine can also cause you to wake up early, possibly with a mild headache. I call this a 'caffeine hangover'. The caffeine in your body has worn off and you are craving more. I fully sympathize with my patients who have this, because I used to get this too.

If you have sleep issues or problems with anxiety, I strongly recommend trying one whole week without any caffeine at all, or at least limiting your intake to the morning. Caffeine is a powerful stimulant. Use it with caution. For many, caffeine is an MSD that nudges you, sip by tasty sip, into stress state.

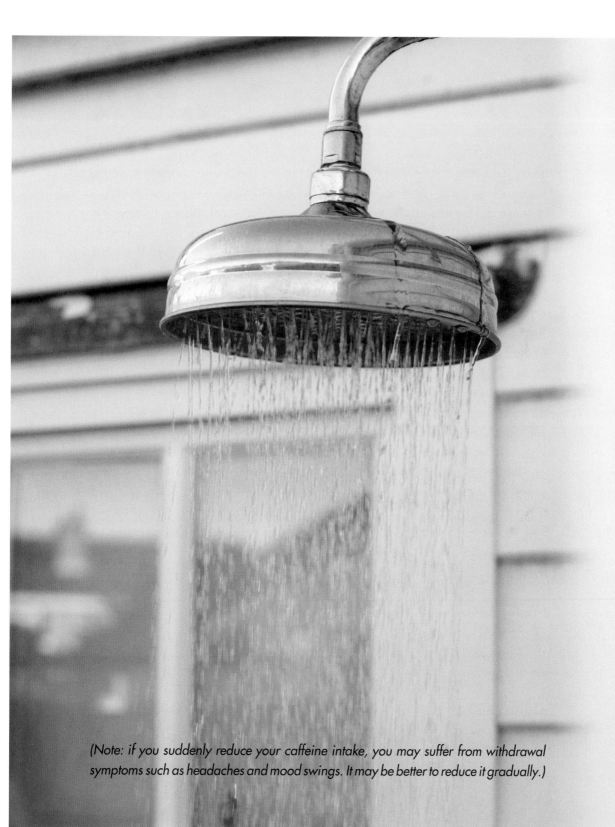

(Note: if you suddenly reduce your caffeine intake, you may suffer from withdrawal symptoms such as headaches and mood swings. It may be better to reduce it gradually.)

THE FOUR PHASES OF SLEEP

There are two major types of sleep: non-rapid eye movement (NREM) and rapid-eye movement (REM), otherwise known as 'dream sleep'.

NREM STAGE 1: You enter this first stage of sleep soon after drifting off. This phase typically lasts up to ten minutes, during which you're easily wakeable. Your breathing will slow down and your heartbeat will become regular. If you wake up from this phase, you may feel as though you never went to sleep at all.

NREM STAGE 2: You spend most of your sleeping time in NREM2. During NREM2 the brain makes room for new memories. By completing NREM stage 2 your ability to learn new things is improved.

SLOW-WAVE SLEEP (SWS): This is the umbrella term for NREM stages 3 and 4. It's a particularly deep phase of sleep during which you effectively lose consciousness and are least likely to be woken by noise. During slow-wave sleep, the brain stores memories.

REM: REM sleep helps you to unlearn and process trauma. Although it is a deep level of sleep, certain areas in the brain are even more active during REM than when you're awake. If you drink alcohol before going to sleep, this is the phase that will be most impacted.

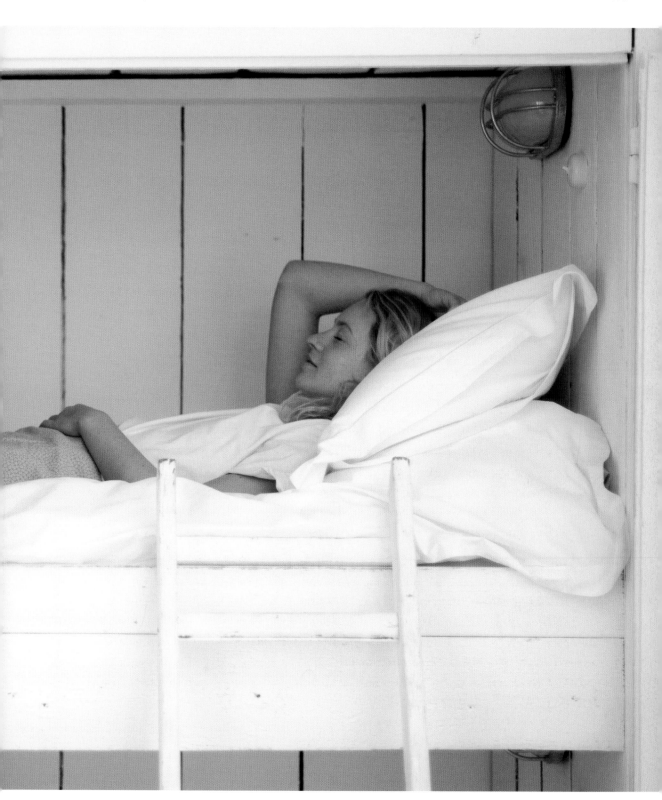

THE SIX WHYS OF SLEEP

1. WHY DO WE SLEEP? Although many of the reasons we sleep remain mysterious, we know that sleep is critical for clearing out the accumulation of waste that occurs during the day. Think of it like a bin man coming round every night to remove your wheelie bin full of physical and emotional rubbish.

2. WHY DO WE DREAM? Most dreaming occurs during REM, a phase in which certain parts of the brain are highly active. There are many theories as to the purpose of dreams, but the whole truth still evades us. We do know, though, that dreaming improves our ability to be creative and solve problems.

3. WHY DO WE FEEL SNAPPY WHEN WE'RE TIRED? When we haven't slept, the emotional brain goes into overdrive. The amygdala – the alarm system responsible for triggering emotions such as fear, sadness, anger or rage – becomes significantly more sensitive.

4. WHY DO WE STRUGGLE TO CONCENTRATE WHEN WE'RE TIRED? The prefrontal cortex is the rational brain's CEO. It calls the shots, making all the sensible decisions. You can think of your amygdala and your prefrontal cortex as being in a tug of war. When you haven't slept well, the amygdala is much more reactive and stronger, which means the prefrontal cortex becomes diminished.

5. WHY DOES LACK OF SLEEP MAKE US PUT ON WEIGHT? Sleep deprivation is linked with obesity for many reasons. Firstly, it encourages you to overeat by changing the levels of two hormones that are critical to maintaining weight. Leptin is known as the satiety hormone, high levels of which signal that you're full. Ghrelin is the hunger hormone, high levels of which signify that you're hungry. Sleep deprivation increases ghrelin, so you feel hungry, and decreases leptin, so you never feel full. This is hardly the best combination!

6. WHY IS IT HARD TO SLEEP IN HOTEL ROOMS? Many of us know that feeling – we stay in a hotel room and our sleep is restless and broken. Why is this? On an evolutionary level, it's because a new place to sleep in might contain a threat and we don't know for sure if it will be safe. Our clever brains therefore resist going into slow-wave sleep, a form of sleep that's critical for replenishment and restoration and our metabolism. It's thought that this is the brain's way of keeping us in lighter sleep so that we can be on the lookout for threats.

TREAT YOURSELF TO SLEEP

If you've had a bad day, rather than sitting on the sofa eating pizza, washing it down with a half bottle of wine and staying up late into the evening on social media, I'd like you to gorge yourself on a generous portion of extra sleep. Light some candles. Read a magazine or a book (studies show that brain activity during sleep is better regulated after reading a book, compared to looking at a screen). Then, when you start feeling the long fingers of melatonin crawling seductively through your system, round it all off with a hot bath. This will lower your body temperature. When you get in, all your blood comes to the surface of your body so, when you step out, your core temperature starts to drop. This is a stimulus to sleep.

Resetting your daily rhythm and getting a large dose of relaxing sleep is one of the most effective ways to take you out of stress state and launch you into thrive.

THE PERFECT BODY-CLOCK ROUTINE

Although it may be challenging to stick to this routine every single day, the more components you can manage, the more you'll be living in harmony with your body clock and the fewer stress signals you'll be sending to your body.

- WAKE UP AT ROUGHLY THE SAME TIME EVERY DAY, EVEN AT WEEKENDS. If you had a late night, I'd urge you still to wake up at the same time but allow yourself a nap later on.

- EXPOSE YOURSELF TO BRIGHT, NATURAL LIGHT EVERY MORNING. This will help you sleep at night by helping you set your circadian rhythm.

- DON'T EAT BREAKFAST IF YOU DON'T WANT TO. Eat if you are hungry, don't if you are not. However, if, by skipping breakfast, you end up ravenous in the evening and eating late at night, I urge you to change this pattern around. In this case, try eating something for breakfast, no matter how little, so that you can reset your clock and avoid late-night eating.

- EXERCISE IN THE EARLIER PART OF THE DAY. If you do vigorous exercise within three hours of going to bed, it can push your body clock back and make it harder for you to fall asleep.

- EAT DINNER AS EARLY AS POSSIBLE, IDEALLY BEFORE 7 P.M.

- CHOOSE NON-CAFFEINATED BEVERAGES such as water or chamomile tea after dinner, if thirsty.

- MINIMIZE YOUR EXPOSURE TO BLUE LIGHT IN THE EVENING. Turn off e-devices, such as laptops, smartphones and tablets, around ninety minutes before going to bed. If you must look at your devices, ensure you're wearing blue-light-blocking glasses or have the appropriate filter on your device switched on.

- IF YOU HAVE A PARTNER, TRY TO ENJOY AT LEAST THREE MINUTES OF INTIMACY BEFORE BED – this could be as simple as holding hands with your partner. (See p. 90 for more information on the benefits of touch.)

- AVOID ANY ACTIVITY THAT WILL RAISE YOUR LEVEL OF EMOTIONAL EXCITEMENT OR ANGER, such as watching the news or a high-octane thriller, two hours before bed.

- ONCE YOU'VE DIMMED THE LIGHTS, REFRAIN FROM EATING. Once it's dark, the sleep hormone, melatonin, is released. In its presence we don't digest food as efficiently.

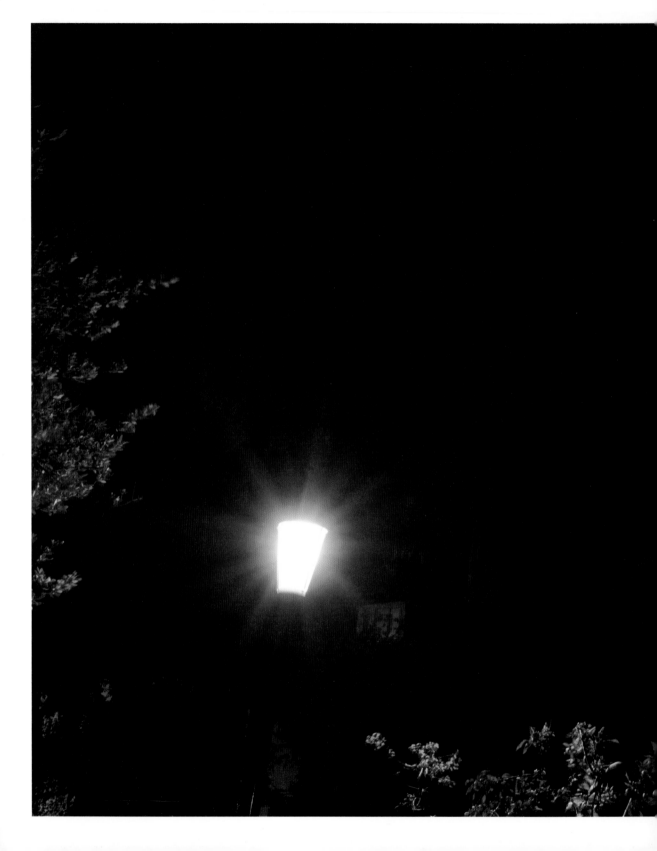

TIPS FOR NIGHT-SHIFT WORKERS

1. **Expose yourself to bright light in the evenings and during the night when working.**

2. **Limit your light exposure in the morning after a shift and use blue-light-blocking glasses to prevent sending your body a signal that it's daytime.**

3. **Exercising before a night shift raises levels of cortisol and helps you feel alert.**

4. **Eating higher-protein, lower-carbohydrate meals,** such as a tuna salad, seems to maintain alertness at night. Try eating a meal like this before you start working.

5. **Avoid alcohol when you've finished your shift.** It will disrupt any sleep that you have during the day.

6. **Try to sleep as soon as you get home in the morning.** Don't busy your mind with lists of tasks to do.

7. **Eat all of your food within a twelve-hour window.** For example, if you work night shifts from eight in the evening until eight in the morning, you could eat at seven thirty before you start, eat during the night while working and stop eating by seven thirty in the morning. This should help set you up for a refreshing sleep in the day.

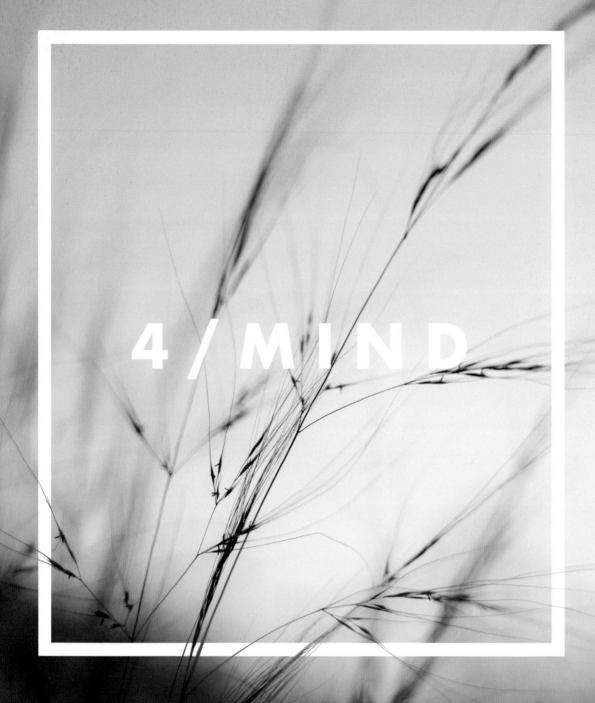

4 / MIND

The alarm buzzer blares. You turn over in bed and fumble towards the sound. You find your alarm clock on your bedside table and open your eyes a crack so you can see what you're doing. The first thing you see is the bright light of your mobile phone. In an instant, you've gone from being in a deep, restful slumber to being in a state of stressed alertness. Does this sound familiar? If it doesn't, you're probably the exception rather than the norm.

Twenty-first-century living is harming our minds. We're filling our heads with stressful information, bombarding ourselves with noise and light. Infinite distractions vie for our attention. We think nothing of continually drowning our thoughts in news articles, status updates, health blogs, text messages, notifications or emails. This information overload is playing havoc with our mental health.

We all know that nourishing our bodies with the right food is important, but we don't think in the same way about nourishing our minds. We need to give our mental health the same daily care we give our physical health. Just as bodies need fuel, minds need stillness, yet the thought of relaxing our minds is often seen as laziness. As I mentioned in *The 4 Pillar Plan*, my patients constantly thank me for giving them 'permission to relax'. I wish they felt they could give themselves such permission. We need relaxation just as we need vitamins, fat and fibre.

In this pillar, I'm going to walk you through some simple strategies to help avoid some of the biggest Micro Stress Doses (MSDs) that are being fired towards your mind. Because overuse of gadgets and the internet is now a global epidemic, much of this pillar is focused on technology. Technology is not inherently bad, but we all need strategies in place to prevent it overwhelming us. I am going to provide you with a roadmap so that you can get the best out of tech without it stealing the best out of you. I will also provide some of the simplest yet most mind-nourishing strategies of all: spending more time in nature and getting into the habit of a short but regular breathing practice.

Chapter 10
TECHNOLOGY OVERLOAD

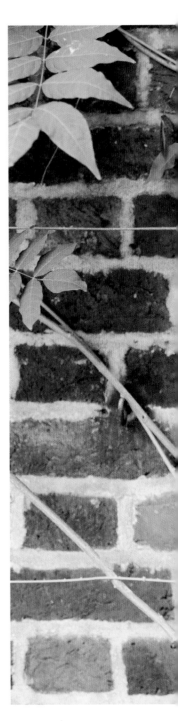

Who can remember the days when a phone was a device for making calls? It doesn't seem too long ago that text messages were the hot new thing, then came the Snake game that addicted millions of Nokia users. We didn't realize it at the time, but we crossed a boundary with that game. The purpose of this powerful piece of technology – the mobile phone – had started to blur. Today, phones are less of a voice-to-voice communication device and more of a beautifully engineered jack-in-the-box crammed with harmful MSDs. You pick it up, turn it on, and they fly at your head by the dozen. That slim rectangle of metal, silicon and glass has got to be responsible for more daily stress doses than anything else in your life. I'm not against the technology itself. It's incredibly powerful and can do a lot of good. But with great power comes great responsibility, and I think the vast majority of us – and I include myself – are shirking it. In doing so, we're primarily harming ourselves.

One of the reasons this kind of tech creates an abnormal level of MSDs is because human attention is naturally drawn to the negative. Our brains want to keep us alive, and it's much more important that they notice and process signals of potential threat than those of reward. But we're simply not built to deal with such constant interpersonal stressors. Humans have evolved to live in

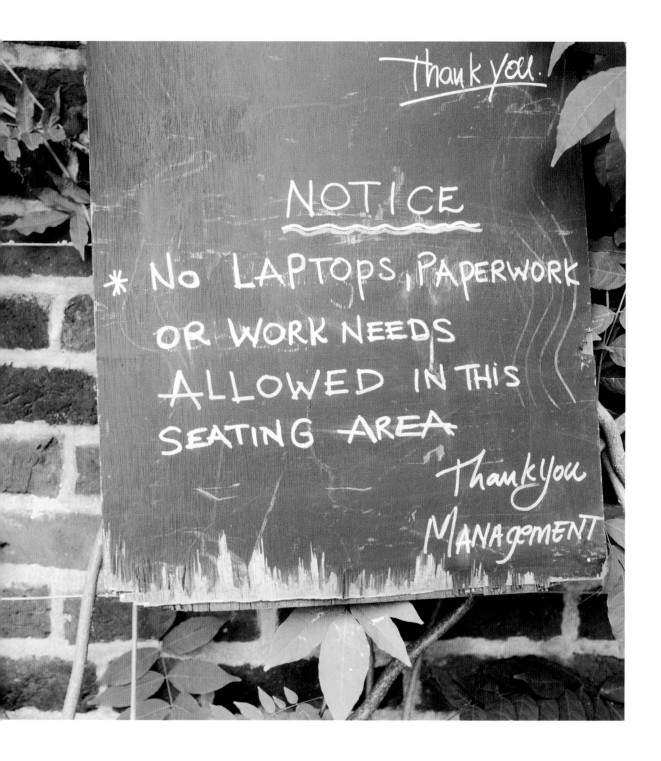

tribes of up to 150 people, yet the average number of Facebook 'friends' is 338. Over on Twitter, the average number of followers is 707. Our social networks are already too big for us to sensibly cope with. Adding weight to this problem is the fact that when people are online they become disinhibited. In a human tribe, interactions would have been face to face, and the ramifications of being disrespectful would often be serious. But now, anyone who's had a bad day can get home and offload their aggression by becoming a brave keyboard warrior, virtue-signalling to the hundreds of people they're connected to.

Put these two phenomena together and you get a very familiar yet entirely toxic situation. When you put a baby picture up on Facebook and receive twenty-three lovely messages telling you what a beautiful child you have, you feel great. But all too often you'll get a snippy comment telling you you're holding your child wrong. Your attention will go straight to that one comment, and that's where it will stay. You'll ruminate on it (see p. 41) and process it for a long time, because signals that something is wrong in your social world are naturally alarming to the brain. It has to make absolutely sure there's no danger in the information. Rumination is another form of stress that's great in short doses but damaging over the longer term. Psychologists know that chronic rumination is a predictor of a whole array of mental health issues, up to and including suicide.

We're never going to be able to eradicate this kind of stress. If you go on the internet, you'll be hit by MSDs. And it's not just from keyboard warriors. There'll always be someone achieving more than you, someone who looks like they're happier, smarter and in a sunnier location than you. Even if you've just been on the holiday of a lifetime, when you come back to work somebody on your feed will be on their own dream holiday, maybe by a pool or on the beach, looking amazing with a pina colada in their hand. Even though you've just experienced something similar, in that moment you'll experience it as an MSD because you're looking out of your office window watching a pigeon drink out of a dirty puddle of water on the roof of a vandalized bus stop. And these MSDs don't simply vanish. They go into you. You absorb them. They change your mood. They change your biology.

FACEBOOK BRAIN

Lots of patients these days are coming into my surgery complaining of increased stress and mental health problems such as anxiety. I've noticed that a high proportion of them are spending a lot of time on their smartphones. I'm convinced this is not a coincidence. Recent studies which examine the effect Facebook has on its adolescent users found it makes them more depressed. Constant exposure to social media seems to be making their emotional brains overactive (see p. 21). I call this state Facebook Brain. Too much time on social media sites starts to change your view of the world. If you feel that everyone around you is having the best time of their lives and you're not, it's going to make you feel as if you're failing, which gives your brain information that it's in a place of threat. If you have Facebook Brain, your brain starts to sense danger even when there's no danger present.

And it's not just Facebook. In 2017 a study conducted by the Royal Society of Public Health surveyed fourteen- to twenty-four-year-olds and found Instagram to be the 'worst social media platform' for mental health. I wasn't surprised to read this. Seeing beautiful, curated images that may well have been photoshopped changes your brain's perception of what's normal and skews its view of reality. We feel we just don't measure up and, again, this gives the brain information that we're failing. I worry about the impact this will have on the current teenage generation. I'm also grateful that social media didn't exist when I was at school. But, even as an adult, Facebook Brain affects me. Last year, I'd just come back from a trip to America and was back at work at the surgery. There happened to be another conference going on that I would've loved to have attended, but I simply didn't have the time. Loads of my friends were posting photos – out for coffee, running on the beach in the sunshine, eating delicious-looking breakfasts. Did I have FOMO (Fear of Missing Out)? You bet I did. Was I stressed by seeing those pictures? Absolutely.

TAKE A DIGITAL HOLIDAY

I'm so convinced of the downsides of being constantly 'connected' that I routinely take digital holidays. Last February I was feeling pretty worn out. I'd been travelling up and down the country speaking about *The 4 Pillar Plan* and spreading the word about progressive medicine. The irony was that, in the process, I was slowly eroding away my own health. In the midst of all the madness I found a few days to take my family on a last-minute break. We went completely off grid. When we got to the hotel, phones, laptops and devices went into the hotel safe and stayed there for the entire duration of the trip. I cannot even begin to tell you how good it felt. Holidays can recharge you, that's for sure, but this was on another level. By the time I got home I felt as if I'd been away for two weeks. It made me realize just how much mental energy is taken up by being chronically connected.

Why not see if you can take a phone-free break next time you are on holiday. In fact, it doesn't even need to be while you're on holiday. A weekend break, a half-day excursion or simply an evening out provides an opportunity for this as well. Often, I will go out with my family on a Sunday, even if just for half a day, without my phone. The benefits for my mental health are immediate and immense – I highly recommend it.

If you feel you *must* have your phone with you for emergencies, why not disable your mobile data services so that you can receive texts and calls, should you need to, without the temptation of mindlessly surfing the web.

In Pillar 1, Purpose, we discussed the importance of doing things for intrinsic motivation, not for external validation (see p. 75). With that in mind, here is a list of questions I would like you to ask yourself:

Do I really need to always carry my phone around with me?

Do I really need to post every single holiday experience to
my social media 'friends'?

Why am I doing this?

Is it because I am struggling to switch off? What purpose does it really serve? Am I doing it for 'likes' and external validation or do I think that my 'friends' really want and need to see it? Am I doing it for my 'friends' or for me? Does it take away from the experience of 'being away'?

My role is not to tell you what to do. I simply want to help you understand your choices a little better. There is nothing inherently wrong with posting a photo from your holiday to your friends. It is much better, though, to be aware of why you are doing it. I have gone through these questions with many of my patients who suffer from stress-related symptoms and in the majority of cases these questions result in them changing their behaviour of their own volition.

THE UNCERTAINTY ADDICTION

Experiences like our device-free holiday convinced me that we all need to take back control from these all-powerful Silicon Valley tech companies. They've spent billions of dollars and recruited some of the smartest people in the world to try to make their products as addictive as possible. The result is that tech is now in control of us. One of their most nightmarish creations is the never-ending nature of social media. The feeds are endless, but we struggle to leave them alone because they trigger our reward pathways. Every time we get a 'like' we receive a hit of the brain chemical associated with reward, dopamine. This keeps us coming back for more. And when we do there's always another article to read, another post to look at.

This effect is magnified by the fact that you never know what result you're going to get when you look at your social media. Is your post going to get ten likes, or a hundred? I know some Manchester City fans who, once the club got rich owners and the team started winning all the time, felt that a lot of the pleasure of going to matches was lost. Every week, they knew their team was going to claim victory. If you know the result before the match has even begun, watching football loses its charm. This same mechanism is in play with gamblers. It's this uncertainty, and the powerful seductive tension that comes from the thought that they *might* be a winner, that keeps them coming back for more.

And it's not just social media. In the past, you might have watched one episode of *Inspector Morse* or *All Creatures Great and Small*, but on Netflix or Amazon Prime you don't even have to do anything and you're already into the next episode of *Narcos* or *Stranger Things*. It's the same on YouTube. As well as being never-ending, these platforms encourage us to multitask, to jump from one thing to another. How many times have you sat down to complete one simple task on your computer and, next thing you know, there are twenty tabs open? All these things are reducing your ability to focus.

CONTROL YOUR TECH BORDERS

I found it fascinating that Dan Nixon, a senior executive at the Bank of England, went public recently, saying he was worried that digital disruptions were having a significant impact on our productivity. This isn't some neurotic GP or a tech Luddite, it's one of the most influential voices in business. Studies confirm that when we complete a task but are distracted while doing it we perform it with an IQ that is ten points lower than if we had performed it without distractions. That loss of IQ is the same as the loss from missing a night's sleep. With our phones constantly at our sides, we're going through our entire lives less intelligently than we might be.

And the negative effect that phones can have on us doesn't stop when we leave work. Twenty years ago you would come back home and sit down with your family or your housemates. You'd eat together, perhaps put the kids to bed then chat and relax in front of *One Foot in the Grave*. You wouldn't have flipped on your device and started looking at work emails. When I ask my patients how many of them check work emails at the weekend, almost everyone says they do. We've normalized this kind of behaviour. It can be Christmas Day and someone can ping you a work email. A few weeks ago someone who has my mobile number added me to a big WhatsApp group. I wasn't at all happy about this, because I'm really careful to protect my personal mobile number. Having someone's mobile number means you have access to them whenever you want. Weekends, evenings, holidays – it doesn't matter. The person who did it wasn't acting with any malice, they simply didn't think anything of it – but that indicates the extent to which we've grown used to the expectation that we should be accessible all the time. We don't respect personal boundaries any more. We steal each other's valuable headspace without thinking twice about it.

But there are things we can do about it. Like all stresses, those that come from your online life can grow your emotional brain at the expense of your rational brain. This means you should erect some boundaries before it – inevitably – gets worse. Taking back control will feed the growth of your rational brain. One part of your rational brain, an area called the dorsolateral prefrontal cortex, or dlPFC, is thought to be involved in our ability to exercise self-control and make rational decisions. People who suffer chronic work stress tend to have a smaller dlPFC, which means they have reduced ability to self-regulate. If you damage the dlPFC, people can be more prone to depression. By controlling the way we interact with our digital worlds, you're exercising the dlPFC and reinforcing your rational brain.

DELAYED GRATIFICATION

Exercising the dlPFC will also help you with a skill that some argue is in short supply these days – delayed gratification. The ability to defer pleasure and reward has been linked to all kinds of positive life outcomes, but in these days of Netflix, Spotify and Amazon Prime, we're becoming used to getting what we want when we want it. We can decide we want a fancy new TV, a new rucksack or simply a brand-new pair of socks and, with a few clicks or button presses, it'll arrive on our doorstep the very next day.

A strong dlPFC will mean we're less likely to be impulsive when confronted by temptation. We can train our dlPFC by taking on tasks that require effort and practice such as:

- Learning a musical instrument

- Learning a new language

- Playing chess, which encourages fierce concentration, mindfulness and focus

- Trying to learn and master a new sport

- Playing cards

- Playing computer games that require skill and patience. (A colleague of mine recently bought her daughter a computer game that teaches dance routines. She tried to play herself and found it incredibly challenging to watch, copy and then learn the dance patterns. This is the kind of activity that exercises the dlPFC.)

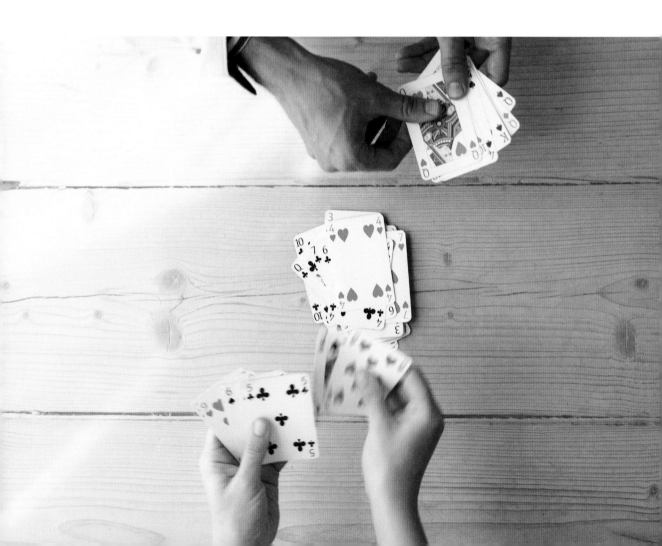

MUTE YOUR DIGITAL WORLD

This intervention is going to help exercise your rational brain. It recognizes that there are lots of amazing things about tech and that it's not realistic or possible to live without it, even if we wanted to. What we can do is dampen its impact on us down to a manageable level.

I'm asking you to pick three of these to start off with. See if you can work your way up from there.

Have a non-tech lunch hour: Turn your phone off and put it in a drawer. Enjoy your lunch without it.

Declare email bankruptcy: This is a great idea I heard from the author Tim Ferris. If you've reached a critical mass of unreplied emails, declare bankruptcy on them. Trash the lot and start again.

Schedule a FOMO (Fear of Missing Out) hour: Give yourself one hour (or two daily half-hours) to look at social media so it doesn't become the default thing you do whenever you're not doing something else.

Batch your emails: Find a set daily time to look at them. Between 2 p.m. and 3 p.m. can work well, because we're often in a circadian lull at this time, and doing more mindless tasks makes sense. Add an automatic response to your email, telling people that you read messages only between these times.

Intermittent fasting for your phone: You might be aware of diets like the 5:2, in which people restrict their calorie intake for two days and eat normally for five. I recommend the 4:1 diet for phones. Put your device in aeroplane mode (or 'airplane mode', if you have an iPhone) for one hour for every four that you're awake.

Mute Facebook messenger groups and WhatsApp groups that are causing you stress: Muting these groups will allow you still to use those services, but without getting stressed. Leaving a WhatsApp or FB messenger group will alert all other users that 'you have left' the group, which may attract hostility or further stress.

Turn off automatic syncing and notifications: Many of your phone apps, such as email, will automatically 'sync', so every time you pick up your phone to make a call you will also see how many new emails have come through; other apps, such as Facebook or Instagram, will send you a notification every time that someone 'likes' or comments on your latest post. Tech companies are like biscuit companies that fill their treats with sugar in order to make them moreish. You can fight back by making sure your phone isn't constantly pinging for your attention.

Open dedicated email accounts: Create a friends-and-family-only email address and turn your work one off during antisocial hours. You can also open a dedicated 'spam' address that you give when ordering products online or checking into hotels so that your email accounts don't overflow.

Put your phone completely out of sight in social situations: Don't underestimate the power of its distracting lure. A recent study showed that its mere presence, even if you put it on 'silent' or turn it face down, will reduce our cognitive ability.

Take notes and keep a diary on paper: Studies suggest that when we take notes in a book rather than on a device we have a much deeper connection with and clearer understanding of it. Why not treat yourself to some new stationery?

If you have an iPhone, switch on 'greyscale' – it turns your screen colours to black and white, which makes your phone a lot less desirable. The first time I did it, the amount of times I looked at my phone over the next few days was dramatically reduced. When I feel that my phone usage is starting to climb, I flip it into greyscale mode for a few days.

Take the news app off your phone: Try to consume less 'news'. I did this a few years ago and it has transformed my stress levels. If you infuse your brain with images of war and the worst of humanity, your brain will start to think that is the norm, even if it isn't. This will heighten your anxieties and stress you out. Choose to consume the news when, and if, you want to.

Track your usage: Until you track how much time you spend on your phone, you probably have no idea at all how much of your time is taken up with scrolling. My cousin recently used an app called *Moment*. Some days he thought he hadn't really been on his phone all day, and the app told him he'd been on it for a solid three hours. He'd touched his phone about every seventeen minutes. The average user of that particular app spends 23 per cent of their waking lives on their phone!

Challenge a friend or partner to see who can use their phone the least: Track your usage on the *Moment* app to see who wins. This is surprisingly motivating. A friend of mine, Emily, does this with her partner. When she is tempted to pick up her phone in the evening she will often resist because she wants to 'beat' her partner. If motivation doesn't work, 'gamifying' the situation can be remarkably effective!

Buy an old-school CD or record player: Two years ago, when I really started to become aware of how addicted I was becoming to my phone, I bought a CD player with no wi-fi connectivity at all, despite the shocked shop attendant trying to talk me round. This has been life-changing for me. I turn my phone off, choose one of my favourite CDs and kick back for an hour or so, oblivious to what's happening on social media or in the wider world. If you're too young to own any CDs, you can buy a non-internet iPod on eBay for as little as £15. If you absolutely have to use your phone, try at least to put it in aeroplane mode.

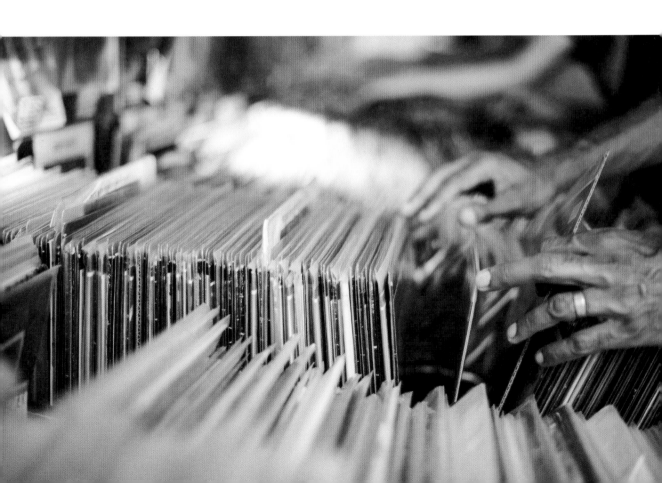

Chapter 11
BATHE YOURSELF IN NATURE

What's the opposite of sitting down and staring at your phone for hours and allowing yourself to be sucked into its vortex of endlessly moving pixels? Nature. Getting outside into the open air is the antidote to technology. Nature is expansive and forces you to look outwards, while technology encourages you to gaze inwards. Being in nature tells your brain and body you're in a restful place, while your smartphone produces an abundance of information that tells your brain you're in a realm of anxiety and pressure.

Nature is profoundly good for us for a simple but easily forgettable reason: we're a part of it. Humans are members of the animal kingdom. We've evolved in nature over the course of millions of years. That's why most of us feel such a deep connection to the open air. I've got some simple gym equipment in my house that I enjoy using, but as soon as it gets to about March I'm not in there, I'm in the garden. I'll go barefoot, do lunges and jumps, listen to the wind in the trees or smell the damp soil. There's something almost magical about being grounded on the earth and in a playful frame of mind. It doesn't just give you a physical workout; it feeds your soul and nourishes your mind.

It's also much easier to exercise outside. It's been found that our perception of the intensity of a workout is diminished in nature. Just think: how easy is it to walk for miles in the countryside, compared to counting down the timer on your gym's treadmill?

There are many studies that confirm the multitude of benefits of spending time in nature, including:

- Improved mental focus
- Reduced anxiety
- Reduced stress levels
- Improved job satisfaction

Results like these resonate deeply with most of us. We feel their truth intuitively. We've all felt that inner sense of peace and wellbeing we get from wandering the lush paths of a forest or playing on a blustery beach. And yet, by 2050, it's thought that as much as 70 per cent of the world's population is going to be living in an urban environment. With increased urbanization comes poorer health outcomes, including increased levels of mental illness. I'm seeing more and more patients in my surgery who I believe are suffering from a brand-new diagnosis – nature deficiency.

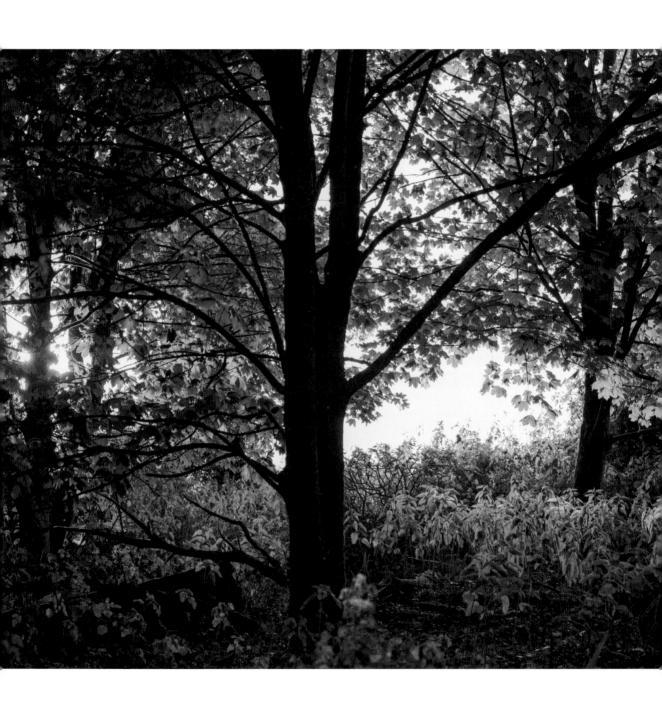

FOREST BATHING

The Japanese believe in a comfort instinct they call *shinrin-yoku*, which translates literally as 'forest bath'. Put simply, forest bathing is about spending time among trees. Experts argue that trees emit essential oils, or phytoncides, which are their natural protection from germs and insects and might even be part of the way different trees communicate with each other. One study of 280 people found that time spent among trees leads to lower cortisol levels, reduced pulse rate and lower blood pressure. Another found that phytoncides can reduce stress levels, increase the quality of our sleep, improve our mood and wellbeing, lower blood pressure, decrease anxiety and increase heart-rate variability (high HRV indicates low stress levels; see p. 169). Another, undertaken at the Mie University School of Medicine in Japan, showed that people suffering from depression saw a reduction in symptoms when treated with the citrus fragrance of phytoncide d-limonene. It's also been found that forest bathing increases the activity of Natural Killer cells, part of our immune system's defence against infection (see p. 86).

Benefits of forest bathing

Reduced blood pressure	Improved symptoms of depression
Lower stress levels	Improved sleep quality
Lower levels of hormones such as adrenaline and cortisol	Improved memory and concentration
Lower blood-sugar levels	Enhanced immune-system function

THE NATURE CRAVING

My wife's parents recently got rid of their back-garden lawn. Initially, we were horrified by their decision. But we were wrong. They decided to create a Japanese-style urban forest complete with water fountain. Just sitting listening to the sound of running water you feel this incredible calm washing over you. The last time I was there I started thinking about all the ways in which our modern, urbanized brains continually crave the natural environments they evolved to thrive within. If we're not building Japanese gardens, we're putting pot plants in our homes, enjoying open fires when radiators do a more efficient job, holidaying by the beach, gazing ecstatically at the stars and at wide views of rolling fields or lying by the pool, even if we have no intention of putting a toe in the water.

Nature helps us put some distance between the 'noise' of daily life and ourselves. It encourages us to look beyond ourselves. Even the simple sound of birds singing or waves crashing can be unbelievably relaxing. One study examined the stress responses of people in a waiting room. Some listened to silence, some to classical music and some to the sound of waves. Those who listened to the waves experienced the greatest calming effect: it reduced their pulse rate and their perception of stress. Researchers in the UK found that listening to the sounds of nature increases thrive-state activation and suppresses the stress state.

Even looking at nature can enhance your recovery from a stressful experience. Research done at the University of Essex has shown that people who are exposed to a nature scene have higher heart-rate variability (see p. 219) and greater thrive-state activation, compared to a group that is exposed to an urban image. Why not set your phone lock screen to a beautiful picture of nature so that every time you're tempted to look at your phone you get a dose of nature? Nature has also been shown to help us break through creative blocks. One study found that when we spend time in nature our ability to solve problems and be more creative improves by an incredible 50 per cent, which will obviously have a positive effect on work-related stress levels. This is thought to be due to an increase in the activity of the default mode network (DMN) that we learned about on p. 60 in the Purpose pillar. In fact, as I've been writing this book, one of my strategies to break through writer's block has been to walk in nature for thirty minutes. Sometimes, just sitting out in the garden and listening to the birds for a couple of minutes has been enough.

THE HEALING POWER OF FRACTALS

One of my personal favourite experiences is seeing golden sunlight flicker and glint through the trees. I find the shapes the light makes through the leaves utterly mesmerizing, and it gives me a unique and joyous feeling. One intriguing theory as to why the sights of nature can be so healing involves patterns called fractals. It's been found that fractals emerge naturally in clouds, snowflakes, raindrops, streams, lakes, trees and along coastlines. Professor Richard Taylor, professor of physics at the University of Oregon, has shown that we're hard-wired to respond positively to these patterns. One of his studies found that we can recover from stress 60 per cent more quickly than otherwise after exposure to images containing them.

According to Benoit Mandelbrot, the Polish-born mathematician who is credited with originally coining the word 'fractal', our 'visual system is in some way hard-wired to understand fractals. The stress reduction is triggered by a physiological resonance when the fractal structure of the eye matches that of the fractal image being viewed.' He found that when we look at fractals even for a short amount of time we get a spike in alpha-wave brain activity which is present when we're in a thrive state. Brain scans reveal that looking at fractals can activate the para-hippocampus, an area of the brain which helps us to process and regulate emotions.

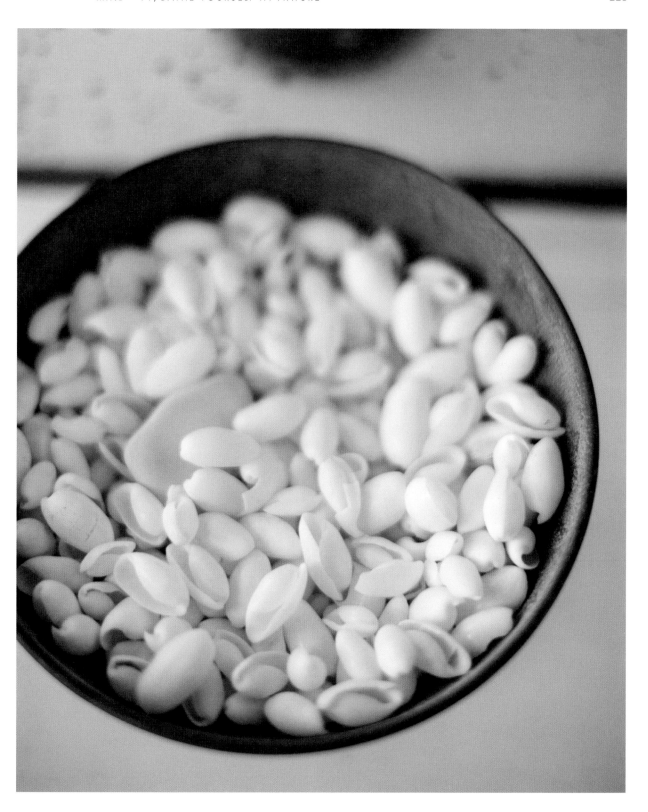

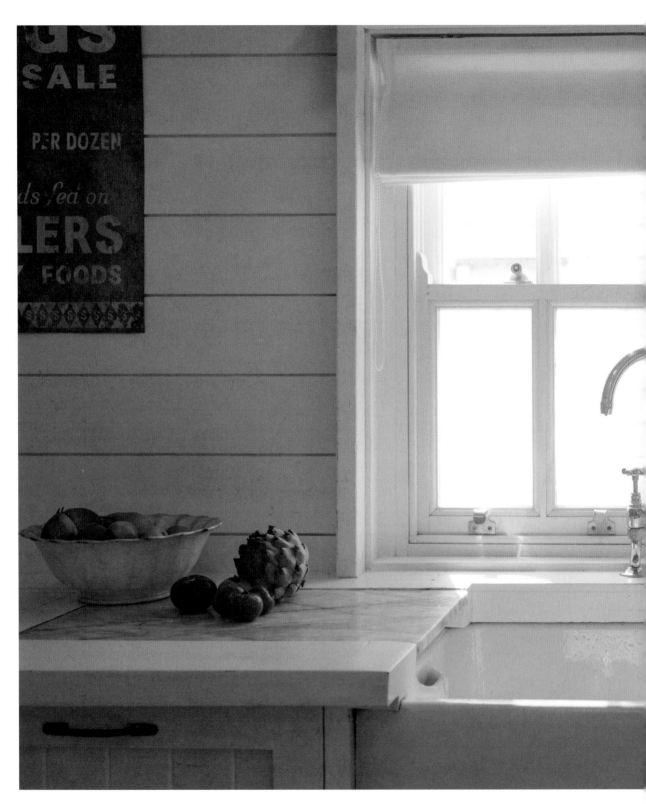

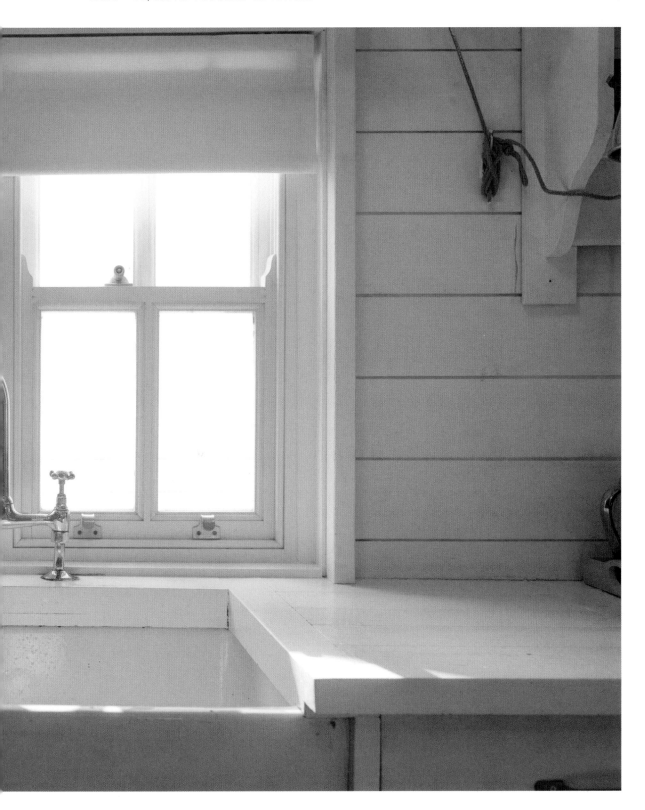

DE-CLUTTER

I once met a guy who'd served with the British Army and had done training in the Belize jungle. He told me that one of the things soldiers learn to help them spot enemy forces hiding in the landscape is to look for straight lines. Why? Because there are no straight lines in nature. I was reminded of this when I visited Times Square in New York a few years back. It's no exaggeration to say I felt almost as if I were being attacked. It's the opposite to how I feel when I'm walking through my local park.

I'm also reminded of my army friend whenever I see a cluttered shelf or tabletop at home and find myself sighing. That clutter is like a mini Times Square. It's an MSD. It's not only giving your brain information that you're in a place of disorder and worry, that clutter will be made up of straight lines and unnatural colours and shapes that are discordant. What's more, studies of brain activity reveal that being surrounded by mess is physically taxing. The brain uses resources and energy to ignore distractions and untidiness. This is why it's harder to concentrate when you have a messy desk or a computer that's crammed with open windows and old documents.

Clutter can begin to take over entire rooms and even houses. One of my colleagues has just hired a new cleaner. He was mortified when the cleaner saw the downstairs spare room, as it was full of junk, cardboard boxes and kids' toys. When he told her how embarrassed he was, she surprised him by saying, 'Don't worry, I see this in every house I go into. Everyone has a dumping room.' So many of us have a clutter problem. It's why a multimillion-pound industry has developed over the past few years to provide storage and contributed to the bestselling success of Marie Kondo's *The Life-Changing Magic of Tidying*, which has inspired millions around the world to de-clutter, including myself. The problem is that we simply haven't evolved to live like this. In *Affluence without Abundance* James Suzman writes about a hunter-gatherer tribe, the San, who live and hunt in harmony with nature's natural rhythms, as they have faith that nature will provide for them. This way of life is entirely sustainable for them and their environment. If there is more food available than they need, they leave it. They never over-consume. They just take what they need. This is how we're supposed to live.

FIVE WAYS TO DE-CLUTTER YOUR LIFE

1. **Choose to keep things that give you pleasure.** This simplifies the process immensely. If you focus on what nourishes you and makes you smile, you will start to give your brain the right kind of information – that life is good, and not a stress. The brain is constantly responding to the world around us. We want to feed our brains positive emotions.

2. **With respect to clothes, how many do you actually wear?** Look at what you regularly wear and what you need for special occasions and ditch the rest. It will also simplify the process of what to wear each morning. Many top CEOs are well known for wearing the same clothes every day to work to conserve more mental energy for the important decisions.

3. **Throw away sentimental things.** Of course, this is only when you are ready to let go. I recently threw out my late father's shirts, which I had been keeping in my wardrobe since he died. I realized that I had no reason to hold on to them any more. I looked at them, fondly remembered my dad wearing them, and happily gave them to the charity shop.

4. **Take photos sparingly.** In the pre-digital world, we would take care over each photo we took. With the advent of smartphones, we take tens of photos each time we want to capture something. Be more mindful about how many photos you take. If you do take more than you needed to, ensure that you go through them and only keep the photos that you love.

5. **Often clutter builds up because our minds are cluttered.** It's not simply a case of clearing out the physical clutter, you need to work on your mind as well. The tips in the Purpose pillar will help you understand yourself better. In turn, you will be able to de-clutter your material possessions much more easily.

A DAILY DOSE OF NATURE

Can you create a space at least weekly, but ideally on a daily basis, where you can access nature? Can you bring more nature into your office or your home? After I've dropped my kids at school, if I've got a bit of time I always walk the long way back through the common, past the lake and the ducks. I've found that if I walk through nature I have a different, calmer feeling about me for the rest of the day. The common is giving me stimulation that's nourishing me rather than draining me. If you work in a city and there's a park nearby, make going there a habit every lunchtime. Most towns, villages and cities have a local park or a canal you can walk along.

Try and access some form of nature each day. Even if you can't make it out to a local green space, use the suggestions on the page opposite to bring nature into your home. The aim is to ensure you are receiving a daily dose.

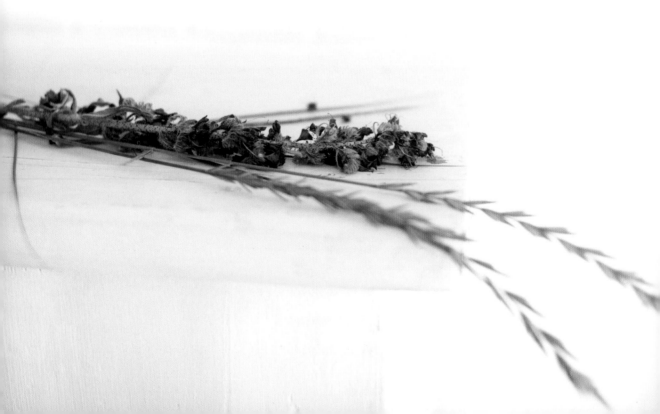

SURROUND YOURSELF WITH NATURE

Below are some suggestions for bringing nature into your home. If you don't like some of them, that is no problem at all. Pick the ones that appeal to you.

- Make your phone/computer screensaver a picture of nature.

- Put up pictures of natural terrain, such as oceans, mountains or forests, in your home.

- Light nature-scented candles. (You could even try reading by candlelight before bed, which will help you relax into sleep.)*

- Consider getting a fish tank or try to create some running water in the garden, for example a small fountain.

- Arrange some sea-shells that you picked up at the beach in a dish.

- Walk barefoot in the garden or in the park.

- If you have no outside space, consider getting a window box or house plants. (You can also save money by growing your own fresh herbs.)

- Before you go to bed, step outside and look at the stars.

- Consider making space in your life for a pet, or offer to look after a neighbour's while they are away. Having a dog can increase the likelihood that you are pulled out into nature at regular intervals.

- Bring health-giving phytoncides into your own home with essential-oils diffusers. My own personal favourites are thyme, lavender or eucalyptus, especially in the winter months.

---

* Make sure the candle is a safe distance from any fabric and that you always put it out before falling asleep.

Chapter 12
TAKE TIME
TO BREATHE

The stress that comes with twenty browser tabs being open at once while all the world shouts at you through news and social media and parades their spectacular lives and bodies all over Facebook and Instagram tends to be felt in a particular way. We can often feel panicky and anxious and our pulse rate seems to soar. I don't know of a quicker, more effective way of reducing this kind of stress than breathing. It's something we all have access to, all the time, and yet so much about how we live our lives today conspires to prevent us from doing it properly. It's as if the modern world has got its hand over our mouths. If you're sitting hunched over a computer at work all day, you can't breathe properly. If you're bending over a screen on the train, you can't breathe properly. If you're wearing tight trousers or a tight skirt, you can't breathe properly. Today's culture puts a vastly outsized value on having a perfectly flat stomach, and the effect of this is that many of us are continually holding our bellies in. Pushing it out is almost seen as socially unacceptable and yet, if you're not breathing with your stomach, you're not breathing efficiently, and this is going to be nudging you closer to a stress state.

Breathing properly encourages full oxygen exchange, and that's been shown to help with a whole variety of conditions, whether it is pain, depression or stress. If you wake up stressed and anxious and you've not slept well, the simple act of doing some deep-breathing practices will start altering your biology and move you closer to thrive state. Breathing is a wonderful therapy after experiencing a stressful incident. It's a way of telling your brain that things are OK, even if you don't feel that they are.

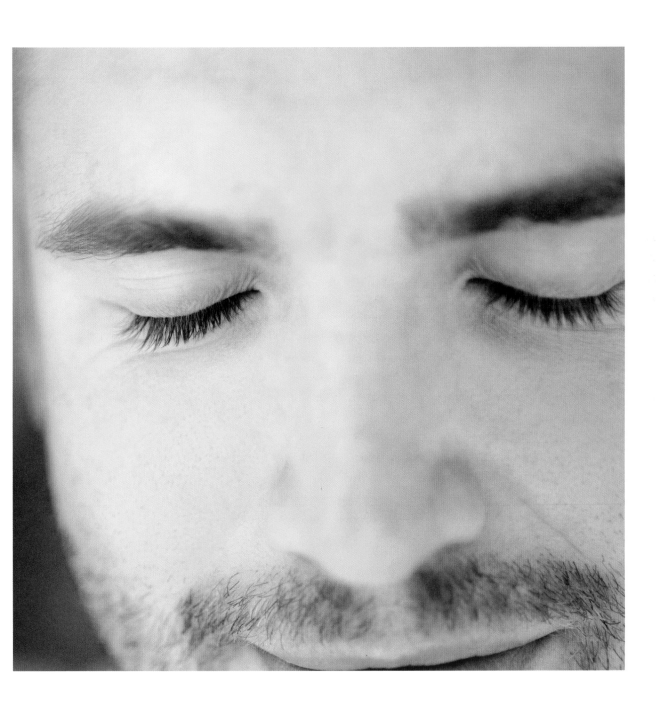

BREATHING IS INFORMATION

Breathing is information. The more stressed you feel, the faster you breathe, and your brain will notice this and read it as a signal that things are not going well. That fast, shallow breathing which happens when you're stressed is effectively telling your brain that you're running from a lion. But the reverse of this rule is also true: if you breathe slowly, you're giving your brain a signal that you're in a place of calm. You will start to feel less stressed. Studies have even shown that the right kind of breathing can reduce our perception of pain. Both the pace at which you breathe and how deeply you breathe change your stress response. If all you do for one minute is slow your breathing down and aim for six breaths (one breath is in and out) in that minute, it will reduce the stress state and stimulate the thrive state.

One of the ways in which this process may work involves a small cluster of interlinked nerve cells that reside within our brainstem known as the 'breathing pacemaker'. We know that a heart pacemaker determines the beat of our pulse. We have known about the presence of this 'breathing pacemaker' that helps regulate our breath for about twenty-five years, but it was only recently that we started to learn more about how exactly it works. In 2017 some brilliant researchers at Stanford University discovered that within the breathing pacemaker there exists a specialized group of neurons that spy on our breathing. Is our breathing regular? Is it excited? Is it panicked? This small group of neurons observes what's happening and then reports this information to the part of the brain responsible for arousal.

To find out more, the researchers knocked out this specialized group of neurons in mice. When they put the mice in a stressful environment, instead of displaying anxious behaviour and nervously sniffing, which is a form of fast breathing, the mice would sit around, happily grooming themselves. This is a powerful indication of just how much influence breathing has on our perception of stress. The researchers believe that, ordinarily, the neurons which were disabled would have detected information from other neurons within the breathing pacemaker that the mice were sniffing around in a stressful environment. This would have sent messages to the brain's arousal centre and they would have very quickly become worried and anxious, as their stress response was ramped up. Without the presence of those specialized neurons, those stress signals were unable to get to the brain's arousal centre, so the mice stayed calm.

Now, I am not advocating that we all remove this small group of neurons from our brain! The implication of this research is simply this: breathing slowly and deeply will prevent us from activating the neurons in the brain that send messages to the brain's arousal centre. We will be giving our body the information that everything is calm.

MEET YOUR DIAPHRAGM

What does it mean to breathe 'properly'? I've always loved singing and when I had lessons as an eleven-year-old I was taught that when you breathe in your stomach should pop out. If you watch a baby breathe, that's exactly what happens. The stomach pops out, which initiates the opening of the ribcage. That baby is breathing as we all should, from its diaphragm and then into its chest. The diaphragm is a muscle that sits beneath your lungs and which needs to expand in order for the lungs to fill completely. You might have noticed this happening if you've ever watched someone sleep. When you're in deep slumber your belly goes out as you breathe in. When we breathe with our diaphragm we involve the lower lobes of the lungs. These lobes, which aren't activated when we don't breathe properly, are thought to have more of the kind of receptors that activate our thrive state, compared to the upper lobes, which have more receptors that trigger the stress state.

This is part of the reason why breathing with the diaphragm and filling the lower lungs with air can be so calming. It's been found that breathing from the diaphragm like this, rather than from the chest, lowers cortisol levels and increases levels of attention and mental function. These are phenomenal findings. If a pharmaceutical company could patent a drug that had these effects, it would surely be worth billions, and yet it's free and available to all of us 24/7.

The breathing process is initiated in a part of the brain called the medulla oblongata, which is located deep inside the brainstem. It triggers the diaphragm muscle to contract, and that leads to space being created inside the lungs. This expansion of the lungs creates a pressure differential which causes the air to flood in. When the diaphragm contracts it moves downwards and rotates the lower ribs outwards. When we think about breathing deeply, we often think about a vertical breath – the ribs go up as we breathe in and go down as we exhale. But the diaphragm is actually a 3D muscle that can move in all three planes – upwards and downwards but also outwards around the body. When you breathe in you

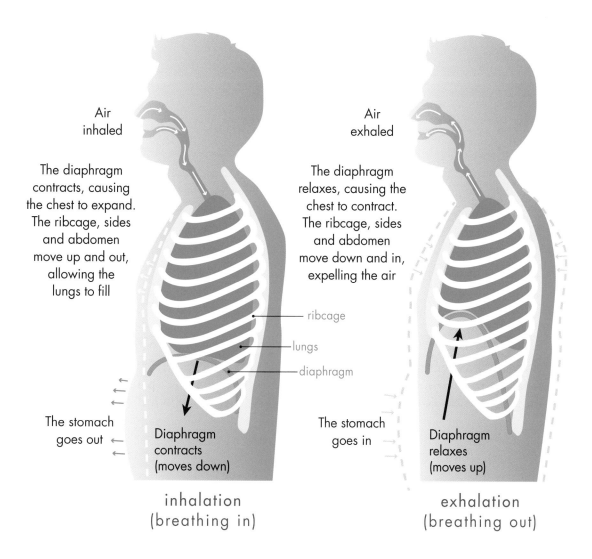

Air inhaled

The diaphragm contracts, causing the chest to expand. The ribcage, sides and abdomen move up and out, allowing the lungs to fill

The stomach goes out

Diaphragm contracts (moves down)

ribcage

lungs

diaphragm

inhalation
(breathing in)

Air exhaled

The diaphragm relaxes, causing the chest to contract. The ribcage, sides and abdomen move down and in, expelling the air

The stomach goes in

Diaphragm relaxes (moves up)

exhalation
(breathing out)

want to expand your abdomen, your sides and your back as well as your lungs. Only then are you realizing your breath's full potential.

When you're not thinking consciously about your breathing your diaphragm will be moving downwards only, and probably by no more than a centimetre. That's enough to keep you functional but it's far from optimal. If we breathe consciously that same diaphragm can move downwards by up to ten centimetres. This is a remarkable difference, and suggests that improving the way you breathe can have a profound impact on the amount of oxygen you're feeding your body.

DON'T PANIC

To understand why breathing quickly and shallowly causes us to feel stressed, it's important to know exactly why we take air in and out of our bodies. Most of us think breathing is all about oxygen, but this isn't entirely true. Of course, one of the central roles of breathing is to take oxygen out of the air and deliver it via the blood to our muscles and organs, including the brain. But an equally critical role is removing carbon dioxide from our systems. If you hold your breath you'll feel an increased desire to breathe, known as 'air hunger'. What many people don't realize is that this desperate urge to breathe is not about being short of oxygen. It is, in fact, driven by a build-up of carbon dioxide.

But, as with so many processes in the body, it's all about balance. We don't want too much carbon dioxide building up, but neither do we want too little in our systems. This is what happens when we breathe too rapidly. When we hyperventilate or suffer from anxiety attacks, or even if we're feeling very stressed, it's common to feel light-headed, to feel a tingling in the hands or even muscle cramps. These symptoms can be triggered by a shortage of carbon dioxide. This shows why learning how to control your breath is so important.

THE NOSE KNOWS

You can compare your nose to a water filter. It works by passing the air you breathe through multiple layers of clever filters. There are fine hairs inside your nostrils that trap particles such as dust and pollutants, ridges called turbinates which help control the humidity of the air, and enzymes within the nasal passages that kill microbes such as viruses. The adenoid glands, which sit on the roof of the mouth, right at the back where the nose meets the throat, produce immune cells to help fight infection. Breathing through the nose is one of the first, and finest, defences we have against the outside world.

Studies suggest that breathing through the nose, as opposed to the mouth, is more efficient and results in an increase in the amount of oxygen we take into our blood vessels by as much as 10 per cent. It also means we're making the most of an extremely important molecule called nitric oxide, which is associated with improved brain function and also makes the blood vessels wider, which makes for better blood pressure and goes some way to counteract male impotence. As well as this, nasal breathing helps the brain cells communicate, improves sleep quality and reduces inflammation. Many prescription medications, including blood pressure drugs and drugs such as Viagra, target these pathways, yet we can access them for free with no side effects whatsoever, simply by making sure we're breathing through our nose.

Breathing through the nose is also anatomically more correct. It means we don't utilize our shoulder or neck muscles, which weren't designed to help us breathe for long periods and can become sore. It also automatically encourages the diaphragm to go down. If all that weren't enough, nasal breathing has also been shown to increase activity in the hippocampus and the amygdala, which is a part of the brain responsible for regulating emotions and dealing with fear. This suggests that nasal breathing could well be a significant part of the strategy to combat stress and increase resilience.

Mouth-breathing, meanwhile, turns out to be particularly harmful during sleep. One patient of mine found he never woke up feeling refreshed and always had a dry mouth, so he took a DIY approach to make sure he wasn't breathing through his mouth by taping it shut! Remarkably, he found himself sleeping much better, which had a significant impact on his health and anxiety levels. A close friend of mine has actually achieved similar results without even having to tape his mouth up. He simply concentrates on breathing through his nose during the day and this has automatically changed his breathing at night. Many people also find benefit from opening up their nasal passages with neti pots, saline sprays and nose strips. If you feel that this is an issue that may be affecting you, it may be worth discussing with your doctor or dentist.

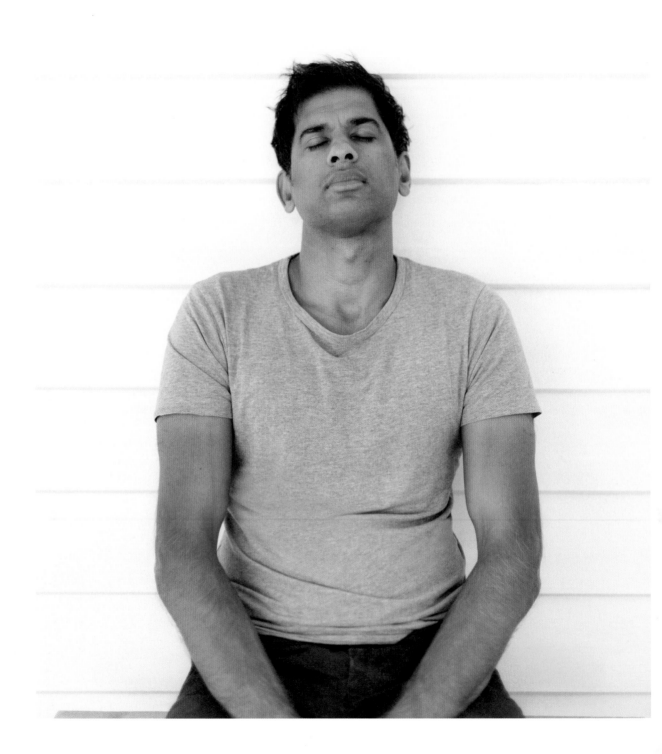

Six benefits of nose breathing

Breathing through the nose may result in:

1. Improved mood and mental state

2. Increased thrive-state activity

3. Better-quality sleep

4. Improved oxygen intake into the blood

5. Better oxygen delivery to the cells

6. Lower stress levels

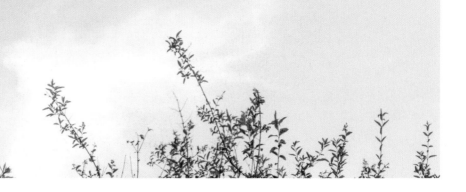

THE YOGIC ART OF BREATHING

Yoga is much more than a physical practice, and many traditional forms strongly emphasize the power of breathing. One Westerner who's learned a huge amount from such practices is Dutchman Wim Hoff, sometimes known as 'The Iceman'. Hoff has managed some truly remarkable feats, such as running 24,500 feet up Everest, swimming in frozen lakes and completing a marathon above the Arctic Circle in just his shorts! He also had LPSs (see p. 139), the incredibly dangerous endotoxins, injected into his body, but rather than this sending him into septic shock, as it probably would you or me, he managed to control his immune-system response with breathing.

Back in 2017 I had the pleasure of seeing Hoff speak in California. He got the whole audience, myself included, to go through one of his breathing techniques, promising that, by the end, we would be able to hold our breath for three minutes. I thought, 'No chance. There's no way,' but less than half an hour later I was not only able to do it, I was finding it effortless. And so were the two hundred others that were sitting around me.

Wim asked us to take full deep breaths in followed by full deep breaths out, each time inhaling and exhaling as much air as we possibly could. After doing this for five or six minutes, he asked us to breathe out fully. He then asked us to stop and not to take any further inhalations. He timed us, and most of us were able to hold our breath for about two minutes. We repeated the entire sequence two more times and, by the end, we were all holding our breath for the full three minutes. You can see a video of this technique on my website at drchatterjee.com/wimhoffbreathing.

Yogic breathing practices can also have an astonishing effect on pain. I have a sixty-four-year-old patient who had been in chronic pain for years and, sadly, took so many opiate painkillers she became dependent on them. When I finally impressed upon her that she was imperilling her life by taking them she became depressed and anxious. She was convinced she wouldn't be able to cope without them. In order to help, I sent her to an experienced yoga instructor.

Today, whenever her pain becomes intolerable, she does deep breathing for five minutes and this reduces her discomfort dramatically. Partly because of this intervention, she's now off the opiates and happier than she's been in years.

ALTERNATE-NOSTRIL BREATHING

Nadi shodhan is one of the oldest known yogic breathing techniques. The idea is simple. You breathe out and then in through one nostril, and then out and then in through the other. See p. 247 for full details. Although yoga practitioners have been extolling the health benefits of *nadi shodhan* for centuries, modern science has been slow to catch up. One small study in 2011 found that six weeks of practice for thirty minutes a day can lead to reductions in heart rate and blood pressure as well as to an increase in lung capacity. Another suggested that which nostril you inhale with can have a significant effect on your body's stress-response system. It seems that breathing in through the left nostril may help calm your body down by lowering heart rate and blood pressure.

These are small, early studies and not of the gold standard we'd prefer for such claims to be considered effectively proven. But this breathing technique has been around for thousands of years, I've experienced a difference in my own stress levels when I've practised it and I've had similar feedback from family members and patients. If you're exhausted, stressed out and running on empty, this practice may well relax you and start giving your body the information it needs to switch you into thrive state. There are no downsides to it whatsoever, so I encourage you to give it a go and find out if it works for you. You could even make it part of your morning routine (see p. 67.)

MEDITATION

Of course, the best-known and arguably most effective form of breathing practice is meditation.

I've noticed that when I meditate I can view my problems and stresses with a lot more clarity. It's as if I've become a detached outsider who can see all the 'noise' for what it really is – often a self-created rumpus that exists mostly in my head. The problem is, that noise can so easily become who we are. Regular meditation can help you remove yourself from the ecosystem of stress you're living in and make you just a bit more aware of what's happening in your life. So instead of it being 'I am feeling stressed,' the experience becomes more like 'I'm noticing at the moment that there's a lot of stress in my life.' This is a subtle but crucially different perspective. Your stress has become something you're experiencing only temporarily, a passing thought, feeling or circumstance rather than something that overwhelmingly defines you.

Multiple studies have confirmed the benefits of meditation in combating stress, anxiety and depression. Other studies have reported that meditation can help lower blood pressure and may improve immune-system function. One found that breathing-based meditation helped people with severe depression who had not responded to antidepressants, another that it can buffer the effects of sleep deprivation. Meditation also helps the growth of grey matter and nerve cells in the brain and reduces activity in the amygdala, which is going to be a huge help for anyone seeking to live a calmer life.

Potential benefits of
meditation include:

Lower blood pressure

Reduced stress levels

Less anxiety

Improved mental health

Better focus and concentration

More efficient immune-system function

Higher energy levels

Less tendency to dwell on negative things

FIVE-MINUTE MEDITATION

There are many forms of meditation. Some of them are breath-based, but many are not. I'd encourage you to experiment with different types and find out what works for you. Apps such as *Calm* or *Headspace* can be useful to get you started, but they don't work for everyone. Whatever method you choose, start off with a daily five-minute practice. Set no expectations apart from the fact that you will sit there for five minutes each day at the same time.

Try to find a quiet space in which to sit comfortably. If it is too hard to sit up with your back straight, don't. When starting your practice, comfort is key – otherwise, you will spend the whole five minutes with tense muscles and be distracted by trying to maintain your posture. If your mind is busy, that is OK. Many people think this means they haven't 'done it right'. This is not true. It is simply a reflection of where your mind is currently at. With regular practice, this will change. Just think, at least you're observing that your mind is busy – yesterday, you probably didn't.

It is important to observe how you feel before and after your practice. However, not all changes brought about by meditation are immediately obvious. Often, the benefits come later on in the day – increased energy, better concentration, lower anxiety and a greater sense of wellbeing.

To excel at meditation is as difficult as running a marathon. It takes regular practice and patience. Don't let this put you off. I am only asking you to commit to five minutes a day. That is enough to get you started, and a low enough bar that you have a high probability of achieving it – this in turn helps keep you motivated. For many of my patients, meditation is the perfect antidote to the stresses of twenty-first-century life and its daily practice has been life-changing. What are you waiting for?

One of my patients, thirty-two-year-old Jenny, worked as a medical secretary in a busy hospital. She found the pressures of the job intense and would often feel anxious, especially when having to attend meetings with colleagues. On a few occasions she was close to having a panic attack. She was understandably concerned about the impact this was having on her job and was scared of losing it. That anxiety and worry in turn affected her home life.

I advised her to take up a regular breathing practice. She selected two items from my breathing menu: alternate-nostril breathing and the 3–4–5 breath. She started to practise first thing in the morning and when she got home from work. In addition, on particularly stressful days at work, she would go into an empty meeting room and spend ten minutes doing one or the other. It made a huge difference. She felt more capable and less anxious, which had a feed-forward effect and improved her self-confidence and work performance. And the treatment couldn't have been simpler, cheaper or come with fewer side effects.

A DAILY PRACTICE OF BREATHING

Take a look at my breathing menu on the following two pages and choose one or two items that appeal to you. Aim to do at least one of these practices every day. Even one minute per day of focused, intentional breathing can make a big difference.

Breathing practice is especially worth considering if you're the kind of person who finds meditation difficult. You don't have to stick to the same practice each time. Play around. Listen to your body. Experiment. I'm sure that, within a few days, you'll find a technique that works for you.

BREATHING MENU

ONE MINUTE, SIX BREATHS. Because making new habits is hard, I want to start easy. For this practice, I'd like you to set aside just one minute to consciously take six breaths. This means that each breath should take about ten seconds to complete, in and out. Use a timer or the second hand of a clock to keep track. If you're new to this kind of practice, you may find that eight breaths in one minute is a little easier to start with. Ideally, I'd like you to do this once in the morning after you've got up, once after lunch and once just before you go to bed. You'll slow your heart rate down, help activate your thrive state and replace a lot of that bad information with good. If you do this for just sixty seconds in the morning, you'll start to become more aware of your breath for the remainder of the day.

3–4–5 BREATH. I find that this exercise can be extremely effective for patients who are prone to anxiety or stress. It could hardly be simpler. Breathe in for three seconds, hold for four seconds and breathe out for five seconds. When your out-breath is longer than your in-breath, you reduce the activation of your stress state and encourage your body to move into a thrive state. You can do a few rounds of this breath or extend it to take five minutes. Listen to your body and see what works for you.

BOX BREATHING. This can be done at any time, but patients report to me that it's especially useful just before bedtime. Breathe in for four seconds, hold for four seconds, breathe out for four seconds, then hold for another four. Box breathing helps lower stress levels, calm the nervous system and take your mind away from distracting thoughts. It's reported that Navy Seals use this method to control their stress levels.

NADI SHODHAN. Alternate-nostril breathing can give a boost of energy as well as help you fall asleep (see p. 241). Sit comfortably, with your shoulders relaxed. Place your right thumb on to your right nostril to block it and fully exhale through your left nostril. Breathe in through your left nostril for a count of four. Place the ring finger and little finger of your right hand on to your left nostril to block it. Release your right thumb and breathe out through your right nostril for a count of four. At the end of the breath, keep your fingers where they are and breathe in through the right nostril for four. Place the thumb back over the right nostril and breathe out through the left nostril. This is one cycle.

Start off by doing ten rounds. You can increase this as you become more familiar with the practice.

KAPALABHATI. Otherwise known as the 'Skull Shining Breath', this forced diaphragmatic breath is a pretty intense exercise but great for a quick pick-me-up. As you take a full deep breath in through your nose, your abdomen will expand. As you exhale, pull your belly button in forcefully and actively, as if it's going in towards the spine. (It can be helpful to think about throwing your breath out.) After each exhale, as your abdomen expands again, you'll automatically start to inhale. Do ten to twenty of these breaths. Afterwards, pay attention to how you feel.

It is always best to learn this one from a trained yoga instructor. Please avoid doing it on an empty stomach, if you're pregnant, have a stent or pacemaker or a history of epilepsy or a hernia.

For video instruction in all of the breathing options above, please go to drchatterjee.com/breathing.

BREATHING IS LIFE

Breathing is the first thing we do when we come into the world and the last thing we do before our hearts finally stop. Breathing is life. It's the simplest human action there is and yet the most fundamental. It brings fuel to the body and mood to the brain. It allows our hearts to beat.

We can't hope to bring our stress under control without first bringing our breath under control. Stress and breath are intimately linked. By spending just a few minutes each day consciously working with it, you'll feed your brain and body the information that life is calm. When you're strongly focusing on your breath you're creating a zone of stillness, a forcefield against which those MSDs have no power.

I want you to stop reading and put this book down right now. For one minute, just breathe. Breathe in for four seconds, hold for another four, breathe out for four and hold for four more. Repeat four times.

BREATHE IN
FOR 4,
HOLD
FOR 4,

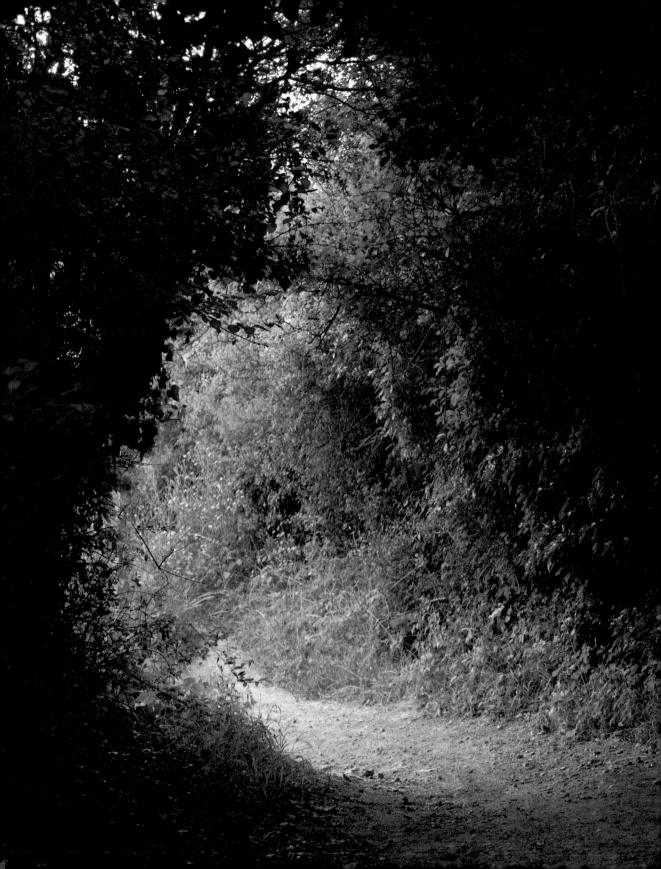